Autism and the Edges of the Known World

by the same author

Sensory Perceptual Issues in Autism and Asperger Syndrome
Different Sensory Experiences – Different Perceptual Worlds
Forewords by Wendy Lawson and Theo Peeters
ISBN 978 1 84310 166 6

Communication Issues in Autism and Asperger Syndrome
Do We Speak the Same Language?
ISBN 978 1 84310 267 0

Theory of Mind and the Triad of Perspectives on Autism and
Asperger Syndrome
A View from the Bridge
ISBN 978 1 84310 361 5

Autism and the Edges of the Known World

Sensitivities, Language and Constructed Reality

Olga Bogdashina

Foreword by Theo Peeters

Jessica Kingsley Publishers
London and Philadelphia

First published in 2010
by Jessica Kingsley Publishers
116 Pentonville Road
London N1 9JB, UK
and
400 Market Street, Suite 400
Philadelphia, PA 19106, USA

www.jkp.com

Library of Congress Cataloging in Publication Data
A CIP catalog record for this book is available from the Library of Congress

British Library Cataloguing in Publication Data
A CIP catalogue record for this book is available from the British Library

ISBN 978 1 84905 042 5

Printed and bound in Great Britain by
MPG Books Group, Cornwall

To my children Alyosha and Olesya

ACKNOWLEDGEMENTS

The largest debt of gratitude goes to the autistic individuals who are willing to share their experiences and ideas in order to help us all learn about the diversity of human thinking and ways to perceive the world around us.

I'm most grateful to Manuel Casanova, Gottfried and Gisela Kolb Endowed Chair in Psychiatry, Associate Chair for Research, University of Louisville, and Professor Geoffrey Samuel, Director of the Cardiff Humanities Research Institute and Professorial Fellow in the School of Religious and Theological Studies, Cardiff University, both of whose critical comments and supportive recommendations enabled me to improve this book. As with all projects, there are ideas and issues in this book that are likely to be modified or corrected when new facts, research findings and observations come to light.

My warmest thanks go to Ian Wilson, a brilliant artist working with adults with autism, who kindly drew the pictures for this book.

This book would not have been written if it were not for my children (who are young adults now) – Alyosha and Olesya. Without them I wouldn't have been the 'me' I am now. Thanks also due to Nigel for his patience and tolerance of my working schedule, and to my three very special friends and companions, Dasha, Lucy and Peter, whose emotional support throughout the project was invaluable.

Last but not least, I'd love to thank my publisher, Jessica Kingsley, and all the staff at JKP who were very supportive of this project. This book benefited greatly from the skills of my production editor, Victoria Peters, and copyeditor, Amy Lankester-Owen. However, the shortcomings, whatever they may be, remain my responsibility.

CONTENTS

FOREWORD

If we could but understand one single flower we might know who we are and what the world is. (J.L. Borges)

When I read Olga's manuscript I immediately thought of Alvarez's foreword to his book, *The Savage God* (1972). Since 'traditional science' has the tendency to study phenomena *in mono* (looking at things from one angle only), he tried to study suicide in literature, because, as Pavese said, literature is a science of life, the one that studies a phenomenon from different angles. This is precisely what Olga Bogdashina attempts to do here. Her *Sensory and Perceptual Issues in Autism and Asperger Syndrome: Different Sensory Experiences – Different Perceptual Worlds* (2003) was an eye opener. In this new book she goes much further in her analysis, hypotheses and suggestions relating to the consequences of the 'qualitatively different sensory and perceptual differences' in autism spectrum conditions. If, from the very beginning, individuals with autism have a different sensory and perceptual development, then it is only logical to admit that they may have different experiences, concepts, intuitions or dreams… that they live in a reality that is different from ours in several ways. Don't they have the right to their own reality?

Olga tries to push the boundaries and explore 'the edges of our knowledge', describing aspects of autism for which there are (until now) no rational explanations, but which have often been mentioned by parents, high functioning persons with autism – 'the native experts' – and 'alternative scientists' in past and present times. Researchers have just started catching up, looking for scientific explanations of phenomena that in the past were considered 'not worthy' of scientific attention. But even now, reactions to very new, alternative or even contradictory 'knowledge' are 'well' (interesting) or 'hell' (don't want to know).

Imagine that all or most of what she mentions is true and that this new knowledge will give us an enormous jump forward in living together with people with autism. Would this not be wonderful?

> To be original implies departing from yourself, from what you are, from your own reality. (Leopoldo Zeà)

If you are 'severely normal' and only want to think and move between the limits of validated knowledge, there is still time to push this book from your table . Yet, be careful. Imagine that all or much of what Olga says turns out later to be true…Think of the recent past where children with autism were still considered as 'ineducable', and how we know now what wonderful persons they may be if *we* open our minds to their differences.

A problem in our society is that we suffer from a cultural superiority complex, and that we think that we, and only we, have the monopoly over quality of life.

Humility, I think, is a core quality: the power to accept that, in fact, we do not 'know' that much and that we 'understand' even less. In a society where autism is not understood well, persons with autism are so vulnerable. Do 'we' 'allow' 'them' the right to their own reality? Are we prepared to accept that 'our' perceptions and interpretations of what is going on around us are not necessarily correct ones (or, at least, the only possible ones)?

In many ways 'autism' is a pilot project for humanity. I do not remember who said it first: 'Autism teaches us about the differences between what it is to be 'normal' and what it is to be 'human'.'

If we are able to accept the differences in autism, then 'allowing' other differences in the diverse population on this planet (colour, religion, etc.) will be easier.

The search toward understanding one's different meaning has to be continued.

One last question: do you see Icarus as a hero or as a failure?

Theo Peeters
Founder of the Centre for Training on Autism, Belgium

INTRODUCTION

What happens when you start writing one book and end up with another? This question arose when I was one-third into my research for the book I've always wanted to write – about autism in the context of spirituality. The working title was *Autism Sensitivity and Its Connection to Spirituality*, and it seemed only logical to start with autistic sensitivities to sensory and emotional stimuli in order to investigate a still ill-defined 'spiritual sensitivity'. It was during this stage that everything went wrong (or shall I say 'deviated from the original plan'?).

I've been researching sensory sensitivities, cognitive and language development in autism for more than 20 years, and I did not expect to spend too much time on covering the main issues. However, I found that the traditional approach, which described unusual reactions and behaviours in response to sensory stimuli and sensory experiences revealed by autistic individuals, was still limited – it did not provide answers to many why-questions.

The search for answers should not, in my view, be restricted to the field of traditional psychology and neuroscience. Autism can help us understand what it means to be human and how we have developed faculties that have shaped our cognition, language and behaviour.

My original plan was put on hold and my exploration of the 'whys and hows' of our senses and the role of language in human life started.

A review of the present research into sensory perception and language development in autism has exposed a very narrow approach. Such a restricted approach limited to just a few academic disciplines is, of course, necessary to deepen our understanding into specific aspects of autism, but my contention in this book is that it is too fragmented and disconnected to reproduce a satisfactory, representative whole picture. All these findings could be assembled to illuminate the whole, but I found there was not enough room in the common framework of developmental and pathological psychology, psychiatry and neuroscience to 'explain' autism and its much wider significance. The context and wider perspective needed could, in fact, be found in many other subject areas, such as philosophy, anthropology, linguistics, biology, quantum mechanics and other sciences.

Uniting the ideas from different fields of research in order to find explanations was a logical step in my research, but unfortunately it has brought unexpected (sometimes hostile) reactions from a few individuals (representing different professional and non-professional groups of people). For example, I discovered that explanations of some of the peculiarities of autistic sensory perception and cognition can be found in the philosophical and anthropological work of the last centuries. However, as soon as I brought this into the discussion, I was silenced by sarcastic statements that Huxley, Bergson and Whitehead did not study autism and per se, their work is therefore irrelevant. According to such 'experts', nothing 'before Kanner' can be used when discussing autism. Yet autism did not appear in 1943 with the appearance of the now famous article by Leo Kanner. It has always existed: either misdiagnosed (for example, as mental retardation or schizophrenia), or 'culturally accommodated' (for instance, in the examples of the 'blessed fools' of Russia, and Brother Juniper in twelfth century Italy).[1]

This narrow approach is unfortunately quite influential in the field of autism. Thanks to forcefully imposed restrictions on how we conceive of autism, rigid and literal interpretation of autism is not uncommon. For example, 'the inability to read emotions is one of the classic features of Asperger syndrome' may be true if we consider conventional ways of reading emotions, which lead us to see individuals with autism as 'defective normals'. If we look instead at the processing and interpretation of emotions in autism from the perspective of recognizing differences in sensory perception, we see a very different picture.[2]

Autism provides us with a different outlook on the same world because the sensory processing functions in autism differ considerably from those of the 'normal' population. This is especially clear in the case of non-verbal individuals. We can establish certain differences in the sensory-cognitive functioning of individuals with autism by studying their experiences, and formulating possible explanations regarding different types of consciousness. However, autism and other related conditions can be studied, and have implications far beyond the limits of medical neurology, psychiatry and psychology. This exploration of the ways in which autistic individuals think and 'see' the world around us assists us in understanding the diversity of our own nature and our own experiences. Autism shifts the focus of our exploration from the practical everyday activities of life to understanding what it means to be human, and the necessity of recognizing the rich diversity of life. Many of us still do not trust anything that is different from 'normality'. We seem to be reluctant to accept that there are many different ways to see the same thing, and each of them may be correct if seen from the right perspective.

There has been a lot of research done to determine at what age children develop the ability to take on a different perspective. For example, Flavell et al. (1981) studied the development of two levels of visual perspective-taking in young children. 'Level 1' is about understanding that the absent person cannot see what the child sees. Children can understand this between 18 and 24 months. 'Level 2' deals with the ability to comprehend that two differently placed people will see two different perspectives of one and the same object. For instance, a three-year-old child and the observer sit opposite each other at a small table. There is a picture of a monkey in front of the child, who interprets it as 'the monkey is standing on its feet'. When the picture is rotated by 180 degrees the child interprets it as 'the monkey is standing on its head'. Only at around four years old can children take someone else's perspective and understand that the person sitting opposite would interpret the picture differently.

Strange as it seems, in my view, sometimes even in adulthood we find it difficult to take the perspective of someone whose experiences are different. We could be in the position of a three-year-old child, who needs help to see that the monkey is standing on its feet. It is time for us to grow up and open our minds to new ideas, or old ideas from a different point of view. This book is not a how-to guide. It aims to show how much we can learn from autism about the world around us, the ways we think and react to our environment, and the abilities we all possess. In the words of Wendy Lawson:

> who can say what is 'complete' and what is lacking? It may be that some of us just view life differently and, therefore, actually help to make up for the 'lacks' that others experience. (Lawson 1998, p.1)

Notes

1. For more information on these and other such examples, see Frith 2003.

2. It is very important to bear in mind that autism is a spectrum condition; there are certain similarities but there are prominent differences as well. Autism does not manifest itself in the same way twice, as there are many types of it (O'Neill 1999). It seems to be useful to view autism spectrum disorders (ASDs) as many 'autisms'. Recent research has confirmed that even high-functioning autism (HFA) and Asperger syndrome (AS) can differ considerably. For example, HFA involves mainly left hemisphere white-matter systems of the brain, while AS affects predominantly right hemisphere systems (McAlonan et al. 2009). There are differences in language development as well. So-called low-functioning autism (LFA) differs from both HFA and AS. That is why statements like, 'we, autistics' or 'my son cannot do it so it has nothing to do with autism' are meaningless.

SENSORY REALITIES 1

Unusual sensory responses (in the past these were often called 'abnormal', 'odd' or 'bizarre') have been identified and reported from the very beginning of official descriptions of autism. Both Kanner (1943) and Asperger (1944) described the bizarre reactions of their patients to sound, touch, sights, taste and smell. Based on their own clinical observations, Bergman and Escalona (1949) put forward a sensory hypothesis to account for the development of autism. They suggested that autistic children start life with a higher degree of sensory sensitivity, which causes them to acquire defensive strategies to protect themselves from overload. These defences, in turn, result in developmental distortions that are reflected in the autistic condition. Eveloff (1960) described severe perceptual difficulties encountered by children with autism.

Creak (1961) included unusual sensory perceptual experiences in his list of the core symptoms of autism. Rimland (1964) emphasized the importance of exploring the perceptual abilities of autistic children. Lorna Wing (1972) included sensory perceptual features in the category of 'basic impairments in autism'. She listed these as 'perceptual problems, including unusual responses to sensory stimuli; "paradoxical" responses to sensations – for example, covering eyes in response to a sound, or ears in response to a visual stimulus [synaesthesia]; a tendency to use peripheral rather than central vision; a tendency to inspect people and things with brief rapid glances rather than a steady gaze; problems of motor and vestibular control' (Wing 1972, p.4).

Ornitz (1969, 1989) described the disorders of perception which are common in autism and extended the notion of a disorder of sensory processing to that of sensory and information processing. This approach allowed him to clarify and identify separate stages and functions in sensory perception, and he considered information processing in terms of discrete functions, such as attention, memory and learning (Ornitz 1983, 1985, 1989). Delacato (1974) suggested that autism is caused by a brain injury that affects one or more of the sensory channels, and makes the brains of autistic children perceive inputs from the outside world differently from non-injured brains. He hypothesized that unusual sensory experiences were, in fact, a primary characteristic feature of autism able to account for the basic symptoms of the condition, then considered to be essential in the diagnostic classifications. According to Delacato, abnormal perceptions might give rise to high levels of anxiety. This, in turn, would result in obsessive or compulsive behaviours, and social and communication problems. Thus these more commonly accepted criteria of autism, were, in fact, secondary developmental problems.

Unfortunately, at the time, all these ideas concerning sensory perception in autism were (unjustifiably, in my view) ignored by other researchers. However, research into sensory realities in autism continued and in the 1960s and 1970s it was suggested (Ornitz 1969, 1974) that autism may be identified in young children if we look at some very specific and easily described behaviours caused by sensory perceptual differences – in the form of unusual responses to sensory stimuli. It was noticed that before the age of six, these behaviours were observed with almost the same frequencies as behaviours related to social and communication impairments (Ornitz, Guthrie and Farley 1977, 1978; Volkmar, Cohen and Paul 1986).[1]

As Temple Grandin argues, the problem is that:

> So many professionals and nonprofessionals have ignored sensory issues because some people just can't imagine that an alternate sensory reality exists if they have not experienced it personally... That type of narrow perception, however, does nothing to help individuals who do have these very real issues in their lives. Even if they don't understand it on a personal level, it's time they put aside their personal ideas. (2008, p.58)

Senses and sensory experiences

Senses deliver information about the environment and our inner feelings to the brain, where this 'raw' information is processed, interpreted and stored for future reference. In the brain our perceptual world is created, interpreted and comprehended, and these processes provide us with ways to act. The connections between the senses and actions are complicated and differ greatly from species to species. That is why:

- the 'real world' and different species' mental images of the world differ
- the interpretation (and the understanding) of the world is based on each species' memory and experiences
- different sensory experiences create different perceptual worlds.

The importance of sensory experience is undeniable. Everything we know about ourselves and the world around us has come through our senses. All our knowledge therefore is the product of what we have seen, heard, smelt and so forth. The process by which we collect, interpret and comprehend information from the outside world by means of the senses is called perception; it has several stages. Each sensory receptor detects its special form of energy/stimulus and transmits this signal to the brain. The reception of the signal in the brain represents sensation (Block and

Yuker 1989). This is an elementary process incapable of analysis; it takes no account of any external object, being simply feeling. Sensations possess quality, intensity and duration. At the level of the perceptual (literal and objective), there is no understanding that things can have meaning beyond what is perceptually available (Powell 2000). After having received the signals, the brain starts interpreting them and makes them meaningful for the individual. Research has shown that categorical knowledge is grounded in sensory-motor regions of the brain (Damasio 1989; Gainotti *et al.* 1995). Damage to a particular sensory-motor region disrupts the conceptual processing of categories that use this region to perceive physical objects (Barsalou 1999; Damasio and Damasio 1994; Gainotti *et al.* 1995; Warrington and Shallice 1984).

The senses

To begin to understand how we sense and perceive the world, we must know how sensory mechanisms are constructed and how they operate to convey sensations – experiences caused by stimuli in the environment. The senses function through specialized sensory organs. Traditionally we distinguish seven sensory systems:

1. *Olfaction*: the faculty of perceiving odours or scents.

2. *Gustation*: the faculty of perceiving the sensation of a soluble substance, caused in the mouth and throat by contact with that substance.

3. *Tactility*: the faculty of perceiving touch, pressure, pain, heat and cold.

4. *Proprioceptive system*: the faculty of perceiving stimuli produced within an organism, especially relating to the position and movement of the body and limbs.

5. *Vestibular system*: the sense of balance and gravity.

6. *Vision*: the faculty of seeing.

7. *Hearing*: the faculty of perceiving sounds.

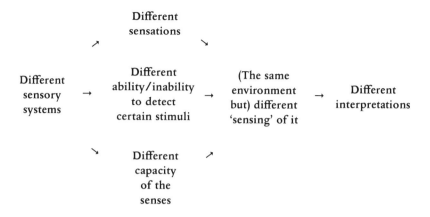

Sense organs transform sensory stimuli, such as light, sounds, odours, flavours, touch, into electrical/chemical nerve signals which are identified, put together and interpreted in the brain.

As we learn to function successfully in our environment, we assume that our senses give us a true and complete picture of what is 'out there', but this is a wrong assumption. The fact of the matter is, we rely on the capacity of our senses, which is, in actuality, rather limited, even in comparison with the senses of some non-human species. Some animals have sensory receptors that are alien to humans. For instance, elephants have special sensors that detect vibrations. Another example is of dolphins and whales whose sonar representation is more three dimensional than that of humans, and allows them to sense almost the entire planet as a three-dimensional object, sensing its curvature (Abraham in Sheldrake, McKenna and Abraham 2005). Even the same senses work differently in humans and animals. For example, cat and human eyes both have rods (receptors sensitive to low light) and cones (colour receptors). Compared to humans, though, cats have more rods than cones, so they can see in the dark much better than humans. Unlike humans, cats have restricted colour perception, but this disadvantage is compensated by their ability to differentiate up to 25 shades of grey (Taylor 2004). Dogs, on the other hand, rely mostly on their sense of smell that is much more acute and has a wider range than that of humans and some other species.

Stimulus → **Sensation** → **Percept**

Each species has developed the sensory systems they need to live and successfully function in their natural environment. Evolution takes care of this. Many birds have remarkable eyesight, dolphins rely on ultrasound pulses that serve them to 'see' their surroundings, bees and other insects operate in the worlds of infrared and ultraviolet, and so on. In a way, humans are blind and deaf to a large part of the sensory universe available to other species, because so many sensory impressions are beyond the range of our senses.

Concepts

Once the incoming information has passed through special areas in the brain, sensory perceptions are joined with appropriate cognitive associations and are bound to general types of things in memory (concepts). For example, the perception of a book is joined with the concept of reading:

Stimulus		Sensation		Interpretation (Percept)		Comprehension (Concept)
A book (an object)	→	A rectangular-shaped object with sheets made of paper covered with printed symbols	→	A book	→	I can read it

As different animals have different perceptual and bodily systems, they have different conceptual systems (Barsalou 1999).

Different experiences	→	Different interpretations	→	Different conceptual worlds

Even if we could experience the same sensations and get the same impressions as other animals do (either via training, drugs or creating complex equipment to 'catch' these sensory impressions which are beyond humans' ability), it does not mean we would 'see', 'hear', 'smell', and so on, the way the species for whom these impressions are natural do. All information received from the senses has to be interpreted (analysed, classified and categorized) to create a complete picture of the environment. And as the 'concepts' of someone with 'ultrasound interpretation' of the world are different, a human armed with the equipment to detect ultrasound but with normal human concepts still would not be able to function in such an ultrasound-conceptual environment. To imagine (and describe) these new experiences we will have to invent new words ('verbal labels') that would convey new concepts.

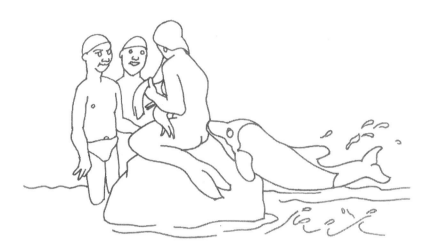

Even humans who have grown up without one or two senses would be confused when their lost senses are restored in adulthood. If one (or several) of the senses is lost (for example, sight or hearing), the other senses develop to compensate and create balance. However, the sensory perceptual worlds of blind or deaf people are very different from the sensory perceptual world of people without these disabilities. It is not enough to shut your eyes or ears to imagine how they experience life. Here we can talk about different perceptions but still similar conceptual worlds. For instance, the blind live in a tactile/auditory/olfactory/gustatory world without any visual perceptions. Their experiences are based on their interaction with the world through the senses available to them. This is by no means a dysfunctional world. It is rather a completely different world. Instead of visual images, they have tactile-motor concepts. Their perception of space and time is different. They perceive distance through time – by how long it has taken to reach or pass objects.

In his book *An Anthropologist on Mars*, Oliver Sacks (1995) writes about a man who had been blind for 45 years and whose vision was restored later in life. A similar case of the restoration of vision in a 49-year-old man (who was blind since he was three) was reported in 2003. Both men found it very hard to adjust to their newly restored ability. They could see, but found it very difficult to interpret what they saw. Without visual experience and visual memory, they had problems recognizing objects, animals, people. As their world had been built up through their other senses they had to learn how to connect visual experiences with meaning. Their experience suggests that though humans are born with visual capabilities they have to learn to make sense of visual images.

The blind compensate for their lack of vision by using their other senses (which often become very acute) and reconstruct a 'visionless' world rich in sound images, tactile and olfactory 'pictures' that is very difficult for sighted people even to imagine. However, unlike severely autistic people, individuals with impaired vision or hearing have the same conceptual world as others. Compare, for example, the experiences of (1) someone with visual impairment and (2) someone with autism:

Stimulus	→	Sensation	→	Interpretation (Percept)	→	Comprehension (Concept)
(1) A book (an object)	→	Recognition through touch, for example, 'A rectangular-shaped object with sheets made of paper'	→	A book	→	I can read it (if it is in Braille)

(2) When I pick up a book, I might turn the pages and sniff each page first before looking at the pictures in it because I believe in finding out first, as a ritual, how old that book is and how many hands have turned the pages of that book before me. Someone else with autism may tear a page or two, for who knows which dominant unit of experience is taking place in his perception. Another person with autism may totally ignore the presence of that book because his perception would be directed toward some other aspect of his environment, and his experience would revolve around that component. (Mukhopadhyay 2008, p.202)

So it is obvious that the real world and the perceived world (i.e. our image of the world) differ. All the information we receive from our senses is constructed (pieced together) in our brain. Our brain cannot process (consciously) all the stimuli present; therefore it selects the key aspects of the scene (defined by our concepts) while the rest of the world falls into the background. That is, the process of perception is an active process, guided by the brain. Moreover, it is a two-way process: information from the sense organs (relatively raw material) is influenced by the 'inside information' (the information we have stored and adjusted to our earlier experiences). Besides, with age we often tend to 'distort' what we perceive even more because we add to our perception by 'seeing' or 'hearing' what we expect to see or hear in certain situations. Feigenberg (1986) suggests that what we see (or hear, feel, etc.) is mostly something we are expecting to see (hear, feel, etc.). The brain does not need to process all the stimuli; it just fills in the gaps and predicts the final picture. This ability of the brain to 'see' before actually seeing is not restricted to vision. The same can be observed with other senses, for example, we can 'hear' or 'feel' what we are expecting to hear or feel. These expectations are based on our experiences and knowledge.

Most of the time, our perception is automatic: when we look at something – for example, a door – we actually see a generalized 'door', not this particular one: we see what we *know* as a door. We do not have to examine the flat vertical surface with a handle every time we see it, to know that this is a door and we can open it to get into the house. A lot of 'perceptual constancies' stored in our brain help us to move in our world with confidence and certainty and save us time for other cognitive processes (solving problems, planning activities, for example). We use our fore-knowledge to 'see' and interpret objects and people we are confronted with at a given moment. As a result, the final picture (multi-sensory: visual, auditory, olfactory, and so on) is inevitably distorted, without us even realizing that our perceived world is not a true copy of the real one.[2] Thus, there is always something of *us* in our interpretation of stimuli. Our response is not objective. It depends on our previous experiences, interests, motivation. Our perception is also influenced by our culture. Though every brain constructs the world in a slightly different way from any other because every brain is different, the ways it operates are similar for non-disabled people. Even with perceptual differences, we see sufficient similarity to agree that a book is a book, a cat is a cat, a door is a door. However, we have to admit given the way we interpret what we see that our 'normally' functioning senses and brain reveal an extremely limited range of reality. The question is: is the 'normal' interpretation necessarily the 'correct' one?

Notes

1. It is interesting that, even in retrospective diagnoses, sensory hypersensitivities were highlighted; for instance, a well-known case of Victor, the Wild Boy of

Aveyron, has been used as an example of possible autism and, among other features, sensory 'symptoms' were prominent (Frith 2003; Lane 1976).

2. That is why we are prone to illusions.

FILTERING MODEL 2

Bergson's and Huxley's filtering hypotheses suggest that the brain protects humans from overload. However, this protective function of the brain does not seem to work in autism.

Some ideas from Bergson's work on perception, memory and intelligence can be applied to the differences we observe in autistic and non-autistic functioning. Though not mentioning autism (which was not identified at the time), Bergson provided profound explanations of some features we find in autistic perception and the reasons why 'normal' people do not possess the 'superabilities' that are quite common in autism (though these 'superabilities' often bring a lot of frustration and anxiety to those involved).

According to Bergson, each and every person would be capable of remembering all that has ever happened to him and of perceiving everything that is happening around him if the brain did not limit these abilities. Protecting us from this overload, which effectively would stop us from functioning, is the main purpose of the brain, central nervous system and sense organs. This function is eliminative and not productive. Aldous Huxley summarizes Bergson's theory in his 1954 essay 'The Doors of Perception':

> The function of the brain and nervous system is to protect us from being overwhelmed and confused by this mass of largely useless and irrelevant knowledge, by shutting out most of what we should otherwise perceive or remember at any moment, and leaving only that very small and special selection which is likely to be practically useful. (Huxley 1954/2004, p.10)

The ability to attend selectively to meaningful stimuli while ignoring irrelevant ones is essential to 'normal' cognitive functioning (e.g. Lane and Pearson 1982). A disturbance in the brain's inhibitory function whereby it filters out irrelevant inputs, i.e. an impaired ability to suppress distracting stimuli, has been called 'sensory gating deficit'. Sensory gating is the brain's natural response to eliminate irrelevant sensory stimuli from conscious awareness (Adler, Waldo and Freedman 1985; Freedman et al. 1987).[1]

Filtering of an infinite amount of information is necessary to make the processing of information effective and conscious. We can only process a limited amount of stimuli consciously, and the decision regarding which stimuli are to be processed in each situation is of paramount importance. What is called impaired selective attention results in increased distraction and diminished 'normal' cognitive functioning, because responses to irrelevant stimuli interfere with the processing of targeted information (Douglas and Peters 1979; Lane and Pearson 1982). The resulting confusion is captured well in these descriptions by two people with autism and Asperger syndrome (AS), respectively:

> One moment you may look at a picture, and at the same time you are aware of the pink wall around the picture, you are also aware of Jack's voice explaining something about the picture. The very next moment you are looking at the reflection through its glass frame, which is competing for attention while you are looking at the picture. You may see

a part of the room reflected in the glass, and you may be so absorbed in the reflection that you may not hear anything more from Jack's voice. (Mukhopadhyay 2008, p.52)

When I step into a room for the first time I often feel a kind of dizziness with all the bits of information my brain perceives swimming inside my head. Details precede their objects: I see scratches on a table's surface before seeing the entire table; the reflection of light on a window before I perceive the whole window; the patterns on a carpet before the whole carpet comes into view. (Tammet 2009, p.177)

We are not conscious of the limitations to our sensory systems (and our 'normal' perception) because we have grown up with them and do not know otherwise. However, 'normal' perception comes at a price – it is *not* necessarily accurate. Let us consider some 'normal' *distortions*.

Recent research has shown that 'normal' perception is not perfect and is susceptible to various forms of induced blindness, for instance, 'inattentional blindness' (a failure to represent unattended objects) (Mack and Rock 1998) and 'change blindness' (the failure to detect large, sudden changes in a display) (Rensink, O'Regan and Clark 1997). These show that the failure to experience some highly visible stimuli in certain conditions is not rare, and is actually 'normal'. The fact that change blindness can be induced in many various ways indicates that it reflects something central about the way we perceive the world (Rensink 2000a). A number of experiments on 'inattentional blindness' and 'change blindness' demonstrate that consciously we take in far less than it seems we are aware of. The research on inattentional blindness (Becklen and Cervone 1983; Mack and Rock 1998; Neisser and Becklen 1975) has shown that subjects attending to a particular object or event often fail to notice the appearance of irrelevant and/ or unexpected items. For example, in the experiment 'Gorilla in Our Midst' (Simons and Chabris 1999) the researchers asked the subjects to watch a video of a basketball game (lasting for about a minute) and count the number of consecutive passes between the players of one of the teams. Although most subjects reported the correct number of passes made by the players, many of them did not notice when a person dressed as a gorilla walked into the game, stopped in the centre, thumped his chest and walked away. When shown the video a second time they were amazed that they failed to notice the gorilla's performance.

The experiments on 'change blindness' provide strong evidence that our attention is very limited. Rensink *et al.* (1997) put forward a hypothesis that focused attention is necessary to see change. These researchers developed the 'coherence theory of attention' (Rensink 2000b; Rensink *et al.* 1997), according to which, a change in a stimulus can be seen only if it is attended to at the time the change occurs. Prior to focused attention there is a stage of *early* processing at a low-level, dealing only with the geometric and photometric properties of the scene. It is followed by focused attention that acts as a hand grasping a small number of proto-objects from the constantly regenerating flux. While held, these 'attended objects' form a 'coherent field'. After focused attention is released, they lose the coherence and dissolve back into the flux (Rensink 2000a). In contrast to an earlier model of object files (Kahneman, Treisman and Gibbs 1992), stating that once attention forms an object file, it continues to exist for a time, even if unattended, the coherence theory suggests that coherent representations (coherence fields) exist as long as attention is directed to them, and there is no or little memory of object structure once attention is withdrawn (Rensink 2000a).

Andy Clark (2002) provides a categorization of responses to these experiments. At one extreme is the notion that our thinking about our perceptual experience is what is known as 'the Grand Illusion', that is, we think we experience and notice much more detail than, in fact, is present in our experience of the world. Though the claim sounds paradoxical, one plausible way of resolving this problem involves distinguishing between conceptual and non-conceptual aspects of experience. This distinction explains the subjective difference between merely thinking about an object in front of oneself, and actually seeing it (Coates 2003). I'd add another level of subjectivity (in our case, there is a difference in autistic vs non-autistic ways of seeing it).

Coates (2003) points out that there are features of the scene that are actually experienced, despite being unattended to: for instance, the person is aware of the other parts of a Persian carpet in the background while his or her attention is directed on to the medallion shape at its centre. In one sense, the person has access to a feature of the environment when he or she is having an experience whose sensory content *actually* involves that feature. In another less immediate sense, the person has access to information if he or she is able to get hold of it – the person has the information *potentially*, and does not need to be currently in possession of it. For example, the unattended aspects of the carpet might still give rise to low-level sensory experience, even if there is a lack of detail.

A possible alternative approach is to acknowledge the role of low-level inner representations of visual input at a pre-attentive stage. Davis, Hoffman and Rodriguez (2002) argue that representations need not faithfully reflect all aspects of the environment. All that is necessary is the gist of the scene to get an idea how to act on it. One does not have to have full and accurate knowledge of the world in order to function. Ronald Rensink (2000a) has developed a theory of attention accounting for a pre-attentive stage of vision. Rensink suggests that it is only at higher levels of processing, where attention plays a major role, that a 'coherence field' creates the representation (involving higher-level conceptual categories) of a physical object in the environment. Before the 'coherent (conceptual) stage', however, there is a 'low-level map-like representation' at an early stage of visual processing. Rensink makes a point that although the sensory information of the whole scene is processed at the low level, little of it is categorized at a higher conceptual level, and that is why little of it is stored in the (conceptual) memory. However, these low-level representations (categorized only by spatial features and location) still play an important role in accounting for changes in attention and in our knowledge of the environment.[2] It has been found that change blindness can be considerably reduced if a verbal cue is offered that describes (in one or two words) the object that is changing (Rensink *et al.* 1997). These results seem to indicate that some sort of scanning process does take place but it acts faster than the process involved in the perception of change (Rensink 2000a).[3]

Would we be able to cope with the vast amount of sensory information we receive if our brains were restructured to let a huge amount of sensory input in?

So we may conclude that 'normal' ('un-impaired') attention is, in fact, very limited. 'Normal' people, in their 'normal' state of consciousness, seem to perceive a tiny fraction of the world they could perceive, if they were not protected by the brain and nervous system's 'normal' function.

As infants, we all experience flooding. The world is in bits, for which we have not yet formed concepts. The concepts bring the bits together. The concepts form our perception. Perception then becomes the key to closing out all kinds of irrelevant information – the stuff that doesn't fit concepts. So-called 'normality' is about becoming 'closed-minded'. (Williams 2003a, p.67)

However, there are people who are born without filtering systems.

Without filtering out a certain degree of incoming information, the slow working equipment of the conscious mind wouldn't be able to keep up with the pace and, unable to make the number and depth of connections it otherwise might with this information, the ways in which we then might communicate, relate, even think or feel, might be very markedly different to what most people think of as 'natural' or 'normal'. (Williams 1998, p.83)

The hypothesis that individuals with autism do not have adequate filtering of sensory information seems to account for the peculiarities of sensory perceptual functioning in autism, other developmental disabilities, and 'normal' functioning in atypical circumstances.[4]

Overload and sensory deprivation

There is an assumption (Minshew 2001) that information acquisition is intact in autism and that the problems start at higher-level processing. Yes and no: yes, because autistic individuals are not blind or deaf (though some may be both blind and deaf, and autistic), but no, because their senses function differently (Daria 2008).

The absence of 'filters' can lead to sensory flooding and may result in self-imposed sensory deprivation with serious consequences. We can outline two different possible scenarios, both leading to sensory deprivation. Autistic individuals' senses seem to be either 'too open' or 'not open enough'. 'Too open' means they have no filters (Gestalt perception – see Chapter 4); 'not open enough' means that not enough sensory stimulation comes through. Both scenarios lead to sensory deprivation: in the first one this is self-imposed sensory deprivation whereby individuals shut down the sensory channel(s) to protect themselves from sensory flooding.

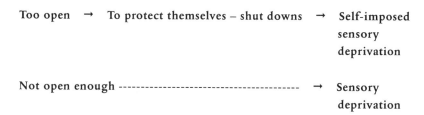

Sensory deprivation can cause immediate psychological problems. Dr Duncan Forrest (Medical Foundation for the Care of Victims of Torture) states that if sensory deprivation goes on for 20 or more hours it can cause long-lasting psychological damage which amounts to post-traumatic stress disorder. After 48 hours of sensory deprivation the effects would be much worse, with the person not knowing who they are and where they are, having panic attacks and nightmares (Forrest 1996), with personality changes including withdrawal, hallucinations and in some people even an abnormal electroencephalogram, typical for mentally ill patients (Doman 1984).

In 2008 scientists conducted an experiment to find out the psychological effects of sensory deprivation on healthy humans. They placed six volunteers into total isolation chambers, constructed in a former nuclear bunker in Hertfordshire, and monitored the impact of sensory deprivation on their minds and physical health over 48 hours.[5] During their isolation the volunteers took to pacing the room endlessly, just to keep themselves occupied. This behaviour is often seen in animals kept in confinement. All the volunteers underwent identical psychological tests before and after the experiment. The results showed a clear impairment of the ability to process information, a reduction in memory and increased suggestibility. Robbins (2008) believes that dendrites (which connect nerve cells) may lose some of their efficacy if not continually stimulated. One of the volunteers described his experiences after 30 hours into the experiment:

> Then I felt as though the room was taking off from underneath me. For the first time, I realised that the lack of stimulation was driving me close to insanity. I felt nothing but numbness, as though I was losing the will to live. I considered pulling out, but I told myself that at least I could comfort myself with the thought that my ordeal was soon going to be over. (Adam Bloom, cited in Courtenay-Smith 2008, p.13)

Such side-effects as hallucinations caused by sensory deprivation are comparable to the visual hallucinations produced by Charles Bonnet syndrome (CBS).[6] Lack of sensory stimulation in CBS makes the brain use other faculties to provide the inner and outer 'environment' (in the case of CBS – visual images are produced).

There were interesting 'post-experiment effects' – the participants' perception of sensory stimuli became more acute after the sensory deprivation:

> When we'd arrived at the bunker before the experiment, I had thought it was all rather bleak. The exterior was all overgrown and the bunker was an eyesore. But when I left after 48 hours, I noticed how green the grass was, how blue the sky was and hundreds of yellow buttercups. It was staggeringly beautiful. Even washing my hands under the tap was amazing. (Adam Bloom, cited in Courtenay-Smith 2008, p.13)

Early sensory deprivation and autism

What if sensory deprivation occurs very early in life? It can be caused either by 'hypoperception' ('closed senses') when not enough stimulation comes in, or by self-imposed sensory deprivation – when a child shuts down his or her senses to avoid painful experiences.

We can see 'autistic symptomatology' in cases of sensory deprivation or sensory impairments, which are often described as 'quasi-' or 'pseudoautism'. The difference between true and 'pseudoautism' seems to be that 'recovery' is possible from 'quasi-autism', if appropriate sensory stimulation is provided, in contrast to true autism where, despite stimulation, there is no complete 'recovery' (Bogdashina 2005). Well-known examples of acquiring of pseudoautism (and recovering from it) are young Romanian orphans adopted by UK families. Michael Rutter *et al.* (1999) followed the development of 165 Romanian babies (most under 12 months of age) in their adopted families. These children had suffered from physical and social deprivation in their home country, where they were kept in orphanages with minimum care and human contact. On their arrival to the UK, the children were assessed and many 'autistic symptoms' were documented, including preoccupation with sensations of smell, taste and touch, impaired development and social unresponsiveness. With the intervention provided by the adopted families, the majority of these children showed a remarkable recovery and were subsequently indistinguishable from normally developing children of their age. Those who were over 12 months old when they arrived in the UK (i.e. those who experienced deprivation for much longer), however, remained slow and idiosyncratic in their development and could not easily catch up with their peers. Is it possible that timing determines if impaired development by sensory deprivation may become irreversible?

Another example is the development of visually or auditorily impaired children. Young children who are congenitally blind display such 'autistic' symptoms as impairments in social interaction, communication, idiosyncratic language development and stereotyped movements (Cass 1996; Gense and Gense 1994). The distortion of auditory input during a critical phase of early development may be one of the causes of impairments in language, thinking and communication development (Tanguay and Edwards 1982). The following accounts of sound perception exemplify this:

> A child with poor auditory perception may hear sound like a bad mobile phone connection, where the voice fades in and out or entire parts of the communication are missing. (Grandin 2008, p.78)

> ...my brain had processed the sound so differently that the human voice was continually distorted. [After Auditory Integration Training] I had now realised that I had heard in surges and troughs, which were further distorted by the intrusion of background noise. I had been so swamped in sound that short term memory and language fragmented so that I could not make sense of my own thoughts. (Blackman 2001, p.276)

Common features have also been observed in the language development of children with autism and those with visual impairments, for example, echolalia and pronoun reversal (Fay and Schuler 1980), and in children with hearing impairments. It is believed that children who are born blind are much more likely to develop autism spectrum disorders (ASDs) than people who are born with normal sight (Tantam 2009). Children who are deaf blind are reported to have an even higher prevalence of autism (Johansson *et al.* 2006). Bearing these examples in mind, is it possible that babies born with overwhelming sensory perception and/or who learn very early in life to protect themselves from painful and overwhelming stimulation by self-imposed sensory deprivation may develop the symptomatology of autism? The timing of intervention may play a crucial part in the child's development and type of autism.

Autism is a classic example of withdrawal. Autistic children seem to be able to turn off one or more of their senses. It can be their protective strategy – when they cannot cope with flooding sensory information they may shut down some or all sensory channels. For example, many autistic children are suspected of being deaf, as they sometimes do not react to (even loud) sounds and many are referred to hearing tests as early as five or six months of age. Their hearing, however, is often even more acute than average, but they learn to 'switch it off' when they experience information overload. When sensory input becomes too intense and often painful, shutting off the sensory channels helps the child to withdraw into his or her own world (Bogdashina 2005). 'It is as though the eyes stop seeing and the ears stop listening' (Mukhopadhyay 2008, p.141).[7] Temple Grandin (1996b, 2000) hypothesizes that by doing this the autistic child creates his or her own self-imposed sensory deprivation that leads to secondary central nervous system (CNS) abnormalities that happen as a result of the autistic child's avoidance of input:

> Auditory and tactile input often overwhelmed me. Loud noise hurt my ears. When noise and sensory stimulation became too intense, I was able to shut off my hearing and retreat into my own world. (Grandin 2000, p.16)

> When a baby is unable to keep up with the rate of incoming information, its threshold for involvement or attention is not great before aversion, diversion or retaliation responses step in, or plain and simple systems shutdowns: nobody's home. (Williams 2003a, p.50)

If not addressed early in life these problems may lead to irreversible hindrance of development.

> In pulling away, I may not have received stimulation that was required for normal development. (Grandin 1996b)

To back up her argument Grandin (1996b) cites animal and human studies that show that restriction of sensory input causes the CNS to become overtly sensitive to stimulation. Animals placed in an environment that severely restricts sensory input develop many 'autistic' symptoms such as stereotyped behaviour, hyperactivity and self-mutilation. Grandin (1996b) argues that the possibility of secondary damage of the nervous system may explain why young children receiving early intervention have a better prognosis than children who do not receive special treatment. If there is no appropriate intervention they may stay at this stage well into adulthood, unwilling and with time unable to leave the 'sanctuary' of autism. (They are often described as the 'aloof group'.) Their world becomes what Donna Williams calls 'simply be' – the world without words, but rich in experience of sounds, patterns, colours and textures (Williams 1998).

Recent studies show that grooming of infant rodents produces long-term changes in the expression of genes. Kaffman and Meaney (2007) suggest that similar effects can be produced by human touching. The effects of early sensory restriction are often long lasting, and the hypersensitivity caused by sensory deprivation seems to be relatively permanent. One possibility is that (at least most) autism may be a type of developmental deprivation syndrome in which disturbances of attentional mechanism (in combination with sensory difficulties) may also contribute to the condition (Blackburn 1999):

It could be that multiple initial deficits (such as impaired attention-shifting, sensory issues, etc., or a combination) could cause a type of deprivation. Attending to only a limited number of stimuli could cause the effects of a limited environment. Similarly, failure to attend to social stimuli or to share joint attention with others could have social deprivation effects. Traumatic sensory experiences may also cause withdrawal or failure to attend, and may cause other effects related to neural over-stimulation, while agnosia-like deficits may prevent learning and association and create its own type of isolation. It should be remembered that even if causing a child to attend to such stimuli were to prevent some of the syndrome, the core impairments would still be there, and it would be unfair to assume that such a child (or adult) is normal. Just as some talented deaf people may learn to read lips and speak clearly, and yet still be profoundly deaf and unable to hear, it is unrealistic and unfair to assume that an autistic person who learns to function is cured, no longer autistic, or doesn't have disability which requires understanding and accommodation. (Blackburn 1999)

The timing of the advent of sensory processing problems may determine which type of autism develops. Temple Grandin suggests the following:

The exact timing of the sensory problems may determine whether a child has Kanner's syndrome [here: high-functioning autism] or is a non-verbal, low-functioning autistic. I hypothesize that oversensitivity to touch and auditory scrambling prior to the age of two may cause the rigidity of thinking and lack of emotional development found in Kanner-type autism. These children partially recover the ability to understand speech between the ages of two-and-a-half and three. [Those] who develop normally up to two years of age, may be more emotionally normal because emotional centres in the brain have had an opportunity to develop before the onset of sensory processing problems. It may be that a simple difference in timing determines which type of autism develops. (Grandin 1996a, p.50)

If sensory problems start early and the child learns to shut the systems down (in order to protect himself from painful and scary experiences), he creates a self-imposed sensory deprivation, which leads to complete isolation of the child from the outside 'normal' world. It prevents him from learning via imitation and social interaction.

Notes

1. The theory of a faulty gating mechanism for information to enter the cortex has been applied as a putative explanation to multiple psychiatric conditions over the last few decades. Not unexpectedly, it is schizophrenia where most of the literature has focused its attention (e.g. Adler *et al.* 1985; Boutros *et al.* 2004; Freedman *et al.* 1987; Freedman *et al.* 2003). The major difference to autism is probably that in schizophrenia gating abnormalities were first ascribed to the thalamus. In autism, the abnormality appears to be in the cortex (Casanova 2009).

2. Fernandez-Duque and Thornton (2000) investigated implicit perception of stimuli by examining whether change could be detected without conscious awareness. In their experiment, they presented two brief displays with a simple array of rectangles; however, the rectangles in the second array, though similar to the first one, changed their orientation. These displays were followed by a test display highlighting the changed item and the item diametrically opposite to it in the display. Volunteers were asked to guess, regardless of whether they had noticed the change, which of the two highlighted items had changed. The results showed that 55% of observers (when the display contained 16 items) and 63% (when it contained eight) were able to guess the correct test rectangle. Though the level of the performance is not very high, it is significantly above chance. Merikle and Joordens (1997) suggest that implicit perception never involves attention. It seems to involve a mechanism operating independently of focused attention; as the performance is better when fewer items are displayed, this mechanism is likely to have a limited capacity (Rensink 2000a).

3. Another explanation of 'inattentional blindness' has been suggested by Wolfe (1999) – 'inattentional amnesia', when unattended stimuli are, in fact, *seen*, but in the absence of attention are quickly forgotten.

4. For a review of sensory gating deficits in relation to the cognitive functions of attention, processing speed and working memory see Potter *et al.* 2006. Though there are very few studies yet investigating this phenomenon in autism, targeting sensory gating deficits in individuals with ASDs may significantly improve their quality of life by relieving them from excessive sensory stimulation and improving cognitive function (Baruth *et al.* In press).

5. Similar experiments conducted in the 1950s by Canadian psychologist Donald Hebb (Brown and Milner 2003) had to be abandoned after some volunteers were unable to endure a complete sensory deprivation for more than 48 hours.

6. Charles Bonnet syndrome is a condition that causes patients with visual loss to have complex visual hallucinations – from simple patterns of lines and shapes (which can be quite complicated like brickwork, mosaic or tiles) to detailed pictures of people and buildings. Sometimes whole scenes appear, such as landscapes or groups of people. These images appear 'from nowhere' and can last from a few minutes to several hours. It can affect people of any age who suffer from failing sight, but more often it affects those who lose their sight later in life. When the sight is lost, the brain is not receiving as much visual stimulation as it used to, and sometimes, images stored in the brain or new fantasy pictures are released and experienced as though they were really seen. These experiences usually happen when individuals are in a relaxed state and when not much is going on around them. It was first described by a Swiss philosopher and naturalist Charles Bonnet in 1760 when he observed that his grandfather, who was almost blind, suffered 'hallucinations': he saw patterns, birds and buildings that were not there.

7. Similar experiences may occur during sensory overload later in life. When the person cannot cope with sensory information, she or he may shut down some or even all sensory channels.

SIDE-NOTES: A FEW QUESTIONS TO ASK 3

Before we start our in-depth exploration of the sensory world of autism, it is necessary to consider a few issues and to ask a few questions.

1. Why do autistic individuals (or individuals with other mental or physical problems) seem to experience 'unusual' sensory phenomena more often than so-called normal people?

Most of the time, 'normal' people know only what comes into their reduced awareness (and through what Huxley calls 'the reducing valve that is consecrated as genuinely real by… language'). Some people, however, according to Huxley, 'seem to be born with a kind of by-pass that circumvents the reducing valve. In others temporary by-passes may be acquired either spontaneously, or as a result of deliberate "spiritual exercises", or through hypnosis, or by means of drugs' (Huxley 1954/2004, pp.11–12).

2. Are the 'autistic unusual sensory experiences' unique to those with autism spectrum disorders (ASDs) or are 'normal' people able to experience them?

Are 'autistic experiences' unique? Both yes and no. There is no doubt that the range and acuteness of the senses can be greatly extended and 'modified consciousness' may be achieved by fairly simple means such as: natural (and/or synthesized) modifiers of consciousness (e.g. some plants, drugs, etc.); mortification of the body, for example in some religious rituals (fasting, lent); meditation[2] and relaxation;[3] illness, fatigue or (physical or psychological) trauma; or even training (examples are vinters, perfumiers and...'stage clairvoyants' who can locate hidden objects by detecting almost imperceptible movements on the parts of their aides) (Clarke 2000). Some artists seem to develop the ability 'to look within' and reproduce the world they perceive on canvas or paper (poets).

3. Is it justifiable and helpful to use 'normal' people's experiences in atypical circumstances to try to understand autism?[1]

'Autistic' experiences may be comparable to a subtype of 'peak-experiences' explored by the foremost spokesman of humanistic Third Force psychology, Abraham Maslow, who claimed that 'experiencing the life at the level of Being' led to the 'cognition of being (B-cognition)' – a tendency 'to perceive external objects, the world, and individual people as more detached from human concern' (Maslow 1970, p.61). According to Williams, Dr Maslow considers these experiences 'valid psychological events worthy of scientific, rather than metaphysical, study – keys to a better understanding of a peculiarly "human" aspect of man's existence' (Williams 1970, p.vi).

However, this connection between autism and the unusual perceptual experiences of 'normal' individuals does not mean that if a person is in a state of relaxation under the influence of a drug, he becomes 'autistic'. The difference lies in interpretation and attaching meaning to these experiences.

Dr Maslow emphasizes that it is important to realize that:

> the knowledge revealed was there all the time, ready to be perceived, if only the perceiver were 'up to it', ready for

it. This is a change in perspicuity, in the efficiency of the perceiver, in his spectacles, so to speak, not a change in the nature of reality or the invention of a new piece of reality which wasn't there before. (Maslow 1970, p.81)

Natural (and/or synthesized) modifiers of consciousness

Hallucinogenic drugs, like LSD[4] or DMT,[5] have scientific interest for brain scientists, especially for those who try to understand perception and consciousness, but they raise very difficult issues as they are dangerous and generally, therefore, illegal (Gregory 1997). As it is a very complicated subject and I have neither expertise nor authority to make any conclusions, we will focus here only on the similarities of certain experiences to autism, which may bring valuable insights into our investigation. Some drugs can produce remarkable exaggerations of sensitivity, making the world appear far more real and vivid than in 'real' life. Yet again, there is no consensus on the status of these experiences. Some consider them subjective, while others are sure that the psychedelic dimension is objective, with each person bringing something to it, but that it cannot be described verbally as we have no concepts which are 'natural' for that world (McKenna in Sheldrake *et al.* 2005).

While discussing 'mind-changing' drugs, it is important to remember the danger and risks they pose. It is one thing when a person participates in a controlled experiment with a drug (like Huxley with mescalin, for example), and another when people start experimenting with drugs just to get 'pleasant experiences'.[6]

In his sequel to *Doors of Perception* – *Heaven and Hell* – Huxley emphasizes the dark side of these experiences – for some people it is the experience of hell rather than heaven.

Similar 'hellish' experiences induced by different drugs are well documented, for example in Thomas De Quincey's *Confessions of an English Opium Eater:*

> ...changes in my dreams were accompanied by deep-seated anxiety and funereal melancholy, such as are wholly

incommunicable by words. I seemed every night to descend – into chasms and sunless abysses, depths below depths, from which it seemed hopeless that I could ever re-ascend. Nor did I, by waking, feel that I had re-ascended. Why should I dwell upon this? For indeed the state of gloom which attended these gorgeous spectacles…cannot be approached by words (De Quincey 1821/1967, p.281).

Dr Maslow warns about using artificial triggers for these intense experiences that, instead of enriching the person's life, he claims, can lead to unhealthy and harmful circumstances as the person may turn away from the world, seeking these experiences just for the pleasure they provide. Very soon, stronger and stronger triggers will be needed to produce the same effect:

Drugs, which can be helpful when wisely used, become dangerous when foolishly used. The sudden insight becomes 'all', and the patient and the disciplined 'working through' is postponed or devalued. [The] valid insight can also be used badly when dichotomized and exaggerated by foolish people. They can distort it into a rejection of the guide, the teacher, the sage, the therapist, the counselor, the elder, the helper along the path to self-actualization and the realm of Being. This is often a great danger and always an unnecessary handicap. (Maslow 1970, pp.viii, ix, x, xi)

Maslow specified when drugs are 'wisely used': it should be 'under observation', that is, part of a controlled experiment. A useful example of alteration of consciousness is an experiment where a 'normal' person, whose sensory perceptual experiences have been changed by a drug and who knows 'both versions of the world', could compare and describe the differences of the perceptual states. A well-known case of this type is that of Aldous Huxley. Huxley was driven to understand the mystery of human consciousness by finding ways to free the mind from the limitations restricting its access to the universe. He was very much interested in science, religion and art. Huxley documented his experiences of taking the mind-altering drug – mescalin – to experience for himself how it changes the quality of consciousness in *The Doors of Perception* (1954/2004) and its sequel *Heaven and Hell* (1956/2004).[7] However, Huxley warns that in some cases, mescalin can trigger very shocking and unpleasant experiences (Huxley 1954/2004). When given a chance, Huxley welcomed the experiment with mescalin, the drug that was considered unique among other drugs: administered in the right doses, mescalin was said to change the quality of consciousness more profoundly and yet it was less toxic than other substances (Huxley 1954/2004).[8]

Huxley was eager to try to experience the same physical environment from the perspective of someone whose consciousness was 'qualitatively different':

> It seems virtually certain that I shall never know what it feels like to be [someone else]. On the other hand, it had always seemed to me possible that, through hypnosis, for example, or autohypnosis, by means of systematic meditation or else by taking the appropriate drug, I might so change my ordinary mode of consciousness as to be able to know, from the inside, what the visionary, the medium, even the mystic were talking about. (Huxley 1954/2004, p.5)

According to Huxley, mescalin 'lowers the efficiency of the brain as an instrument for focusing the mind on the problems of' everyday life and permits 'the entry into consciousness of certain classes of mental events, which are normally excluded, because they possess no survival value' (Huxley 1956/2004, p.57). Huxley shows the effects of mescalin on brain functioning (which do not include the interference in intellectual functioning) as follows:

> The ability to remember and to 'think straight' is little if at all reduced…[unlike under the influence of alcohol]. Visual impressions are greatly intensified and the eye recovers some of the perceptual innocence of childhood, when the sensum was not immediately and automatically subordinated to the concept. (Huxley 1954/2004, p.12)

There are some side-effects of mescalin, such as, for example, withdrawal and loss of interest in the outside world, while:

> [the] ego grows weak, he can't be bothered to undertake the necessary chores, and loses all interest in those spatial and temporal relationships which mean so much to an organism bent on getting on in the world. As Mind at Large seeps past the no longer watertight valve, all kind of biologically useless things start to happen. In some cases there may be extra-sensory perceptions. Other persons discover a world of visionary beauty. To others again is revealed the glory, the infinite value and meaningfulness of naked existence, of the given, unconceptualized event. In the final stage of egolessness there is an 'obscure knowledge' that All is in all – that All is actually each. (Huxley 1954/2004, pp.11–12)

Huxley (1954/2004) hypothesizes that mescalin seems to have a power to impair the efficiency of the cerebral reducing valve (reducing filtering ability) and to bring forth 'cleansed perception'. The experiences of non-autistic people, like Huxley, for example, and high-functioning autistic individuals who can articulate them, can help us understand the abilities and problems of those non-verbal autistic individuals who struggle to communicate their differences.

It is important to remember that the experiences induced by chemicals or chemical changes in the body last only for a few hours. People involved just 'visit' a 'different sensory perceptual world' as tourists visiting a different culture while maintaining their own. However, there are people who are born and grow up in 'different perceptual worlds', for whom the different 'language-less') world of 'Being'/'Is-ness' is home. For autistic individuals, for example, this unconceptualized 'world' is the one they were born into. Some can develop abilities to leave it (even if temporarily) to visit the world of the majority, but some never get a visa to cross the border and they stay in their world most of their lives:

> It had been the same as long as I had known…some things hadn't changed…since I was an infant swept up in the

perception of swirling air particles, a child lost in repetition of a pattern of sound, or a teenager staring for hours at coloured billiard balls, trying to grasp the experience of the particular colour I was climbing into. (Williams 1999a, p.19)

Notes

1. I apologize if anyone would find themselves offended by the suggestion that a drug-induced state of consciousness gives an insight into the abilities and problems of those non-verbal autistic individuals who struggle to communicate their differences.

2. In Tibetan tradition the process of self-cultivation is conceived, among other things, in terms of internal flows, currents or winds. One has to learn to control the flows (*prana* in Sanskrit, *lung* in Tibetan – both encompassing cognitive, emotional and volitional states) through physical exercises and internal visualizations. What is often classified as 'psychiatric illness' in Western medicine is seen in Tibetan medical practice as 'lung imbalance'. Much of the specifically religious imagery of Buddhism can be of relevance to some people with ASDs (Samuel 2009).

3. Similar experiences (though rare) can be achieved in a relaxed brain state; for example, consider the experience of an American scientist, C. King, who was waiting on a New Jersey railway platform:

   Suddenly the entire aspect of the surroundings changed. The whole atmosphere seemed strangely vitalized and abruptly the few other persons on the platform took on an appearance hardly more important or significant than that of the doorknobs at the entrance to the passengers' waiting room. But the most extraordinary alteration was that of the dun-coloured bricks. They remained, naturally, dun-coloured bricks, for there was no concomitant sensory illusion in the experience. But all at once they appeared to be tremendously alive: without manifesting any exterior motion they seemed to be seething almost joyously inside and gave the distinct impression that in their own degree they were living and actively liking it. (King 1963, p.120)

4. In LSD, or lysergic acid diethylamide, the lysergic acid component is derived from ergot, a wild fungus. LSD works by interfering with the thalamus – the part of the brain that interprets sights, smells and sounds. A 'trip' lasts about 12 hours and can boost levels of serotonin in the brain. When these levels drop, the user experiences a come-down. Some users experience a 'bad trip' and feel terrified. LSD was discovered by Albert Hoffman, Swiss chemist, in 1938. The discovery was incidental but had

huge consequences. In the 1960s, LSD began to be used first as a pathway to spiritual enlightenment, and then as a recreational drug. Though it was originally believed to be a 'wonder drug', the decades of its being available have shown that if it is 'foolishly used' (to borrow Maslow's terms), LSD is dangerous and unpredictable; it may lead to erratic and fatal behaviour, such as, for example, a belief the user can fly. The fact that it became cheap and easily available left it open to abuse. After a number of people committed suicide after its influence, LSD was banned around the world. The son of 1960s cult psychiatrist, R.D. Laing, who regularly took the drug himself and championed the use of LSD with his patients, committed suicide at the age of 40 under the influence of drugs.

5. DMT is a psychoactive chemical that is naturally found in the human body in small quantities, and also in many plants; it causes intense visions as if the user has entered a completely different 'world' that some consider a parallel universe – 'DMTverse' (Pickover 2005). For example, author Terence McKenna, who experimented with DMT, feels that 'right here and now, one quanta away, there is raging a universe of active intelligence that is transhuman, hyperdimensional, and extremely alien… What is driving religious feeling today is a wish for contact with this universe' (McKenna 1992, p.38). DMT is a dangerous drug which is open to abuse and has no medical value.

6. There is no consensus in relation to the legality or illegality of psychedelic drugs: some believe that psychedelics can be used to explore the potential of the human mind, while others strongly oppose the availability and usage of any psychedelics. The consequences (even if for a minority) can be horrendous and many lives have been destroyed.

7. According to Huxley (1954/2004), mescalin is the active principle of peyote, a root of the plant, which the Indians of Mexico and the American Southwest venerate as though it were a deity. According to Huxley mescalin (unlike other drugs) is not addictive: its effects will disappear after eight or ten hours and there is no craving for it. Professor J.S. Slotkin, who studied and participated in the rites of a Peyotist congregation, testified that his fellow worshippers certainly were not drunk or stupefied. He described them as quiet, courteous and considerate towards one another (Huxley 1954/2004, p.44).

8. Huxley points out the similarity in chemical composition between mescalin and adrenalin: the product of decomposition of adrenalin (adrenochrome), which is natural for the human body, can produce similar symptoms to those caused by mescalin intoxication. Thus, Huxley argues, each of us is capable of producing a chemical that can cause profound alterations of consciousness. Some of these changes can be observed in schizophrenia.

GESTALT PERCEPTION 4

The most striking feature of many autistic individuals' perception is that their senses are 'too open', and incoming information is not filtered or selected. All the stimuli are perceived simultaneously (at the stage of sensation, without awareness of concepts). This is known as Gestalt perception (Bogdashina 2003) and seems to be caused by 'sensory gating deficit'. Things are just patterns of sensory stimuli, not functional objects. Due to Gestalt perception autistic children may exhibit delayed concept acquisition that, in turn, slows down the development of verbal language. During the 'concept-less' period they seem to have difficulty learning the conventional functions of objects around them. That is just how Huxley describes the concept-less (Gestalt) experience under the influence of mescalin:

> A small typing table stood in the center of the room; beyond it…was a wicker chair and beyond that a desk. The three pieces formed an intricate pattern of horizontals, uprights and diagonals – a pattern all the more interesting for not being interpreted in terms of spatial relationships. Table, chair and desk came together in a composition that was like something by Braque or Juan Gris, a still life recognizably

related to the objective world, but rendered without depth, without any attempt at photographic realism. I was looking at my furniture, not as the utilitarian who has to sit on chairs, to write at desks and tables, and not as the cameraman or scientific recorder, but as the pure aesthete whose concern is only with forms and their relationships within the field of vision or the picture of space. (Huxley 1954/2004, pp.9–10)

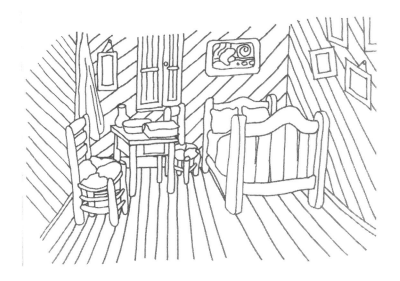

Unlike those so-called low-functioning autistic individuals who never experience what it is like for 'normal' people, Huxley actually knew the 'conventional' conceptualized world and experienced the confusing 'concept-less' state only for a few hours:

> For what seemed an immensely long time I gazed without knowing, even without wishing to know, what it was that confronted me. At any other time I would have seen a chair barred with alternate light and shade. Today the percept had swallowed up the concept. I was so completely absorbed in looking, so thunderstruck by what I actually saw, that I could not be aware of anything else. (Huxley 1954/2004, p.32)

Maslow describes cognitive function in similar peak-experiences as follows:

> In the cognition that comes in peak-experiences, characteristically the percept is exclusively and fully attended to. That is, there is tremendous concentration of a kind which does not normally occur. There is the truest and most total kind of visual perceiving or listening or feeling. Part of what this involves is a peculiar change which can be best described as non-evaluating, non-comparing, or non-judging cognition. [F]igures and ground are less sharply differentiated...there is a tendency for things to become equally important rather than to be ranged in a hierarchy from very important to quite important. (Maslow 1970, p.60)

For many autistic individuals the inability to or difficulty with filtering incoming stimuli can be overwhelming. For example, once, on being invited to a reception party in Los Angeles, Tito found himself in a crowded room, which had a high ceiling, many doors, and several pictures on the walls, where every corner seemed to demand his attention; colours and voices competed with each other, making it hard to focus on anything (Mukhopadhyay 2008).

The research of UCSF (University of California, San Francisco) neuroscientist Michael Merzenich and neurogeneticist John Rubenstein has suggested that there seems to be a disproportionately high level of excitation (or disproportionately weak inhibition) in the sensory, mnemonic, social and emotional systems of autistic individuals (Rubenstein and Merzenich 2003). These researchers also studied the effects of auditory bombardment on developing brains. In experiments with rats whose developing forebrains were exposed to sequenced bursts of noise at different frequencies (simulating inherited genetic weakness in humans), they found that the 'critical period' ended too early. The brains had not developed, in time, a full repertoire of the circuits which underlie perception, memory, and cognitive and language abilities. In related experiments, rats were subjected to continuous, nonpulsating sound (similar to white noise) and the same problem emerged, if for a different reason – the critical period window stayed open too long. As a result differentiation was delayed indefinitely, leaving the rats' brains more susceptible to cortical epilepsy. Merzenich hypothesizes that both scenarios could explain autism. In both of these hypothetical 'noisy processing' developmental scenarios, the auditory speech cortex would mature through the critical period of development and enter the 'adult' epoch in a highly undifferentiated and relatively unstable state (Rubenstein and Merzenich 2003).

Such studies indicate that the auditory environment has a paramount impact on the progression of the fundamental maturation and specialization of the primary auditory cortex, and implicate a number of specific sensory factors that could potentially amplify or otherwise modulate developmental progressions (Rubenstein and Merzenich 2003). It has been suggested that altered inhibitory control of sensory intake in autism may cause sensory overload leading to avoidance of external stimulation (Khalfa *et al.* 2004). Similar problems have been reported in early visual processing. Baruth *et al.* (In press) investigated cortical responses elicited by task-irrelevant visual stimuli in individuals with autism and age-matched typically developing control subjects. The participants with autism spectrum disorder (ASD) failed to suppress cortical responses at early stages of visual processing and significantly underperformed with respect to the controls in target stimulus detection. These results indicate a visual gating deficit in ASD.

Merzenich's research highlights the importance of the 'sound quality', particularly in childrearing environments. It turns out to be true to other senses as well. The Markrams' 'intense world hypothesis' shows that in order to help babies at risk (those whose senses are hypersensitive and whose filtering does not work properly) we have to protect them from 'sensory assault', so typical of our time. The majority of the population seems to have a very high sensory threshold and inhabits an ever louder, brighter, smellier, and so forth environment. Babies are exposed to a blaring television, loud music, blasting radio, ringing phones, fluorescent lights. The world of the majority has become desensitized, and needs higher stimulation to notice sensations. It leaves the vulnerable minority, not equipped with filtering systems, in a constant struggle to survive a kind of 'sensory torture'. Instead of protecting them, we expose them from early life to excessive overstimulation:

> Today's fast paced, techno-driven world is louder and busier than the world I grew up in. That, in and of itself, creates new challenges for the child with autism, whose sensory systems are usually impaired in one way or another. Our senses are bombarded on a daily basis, and this can render even typical children and adults exhausted by the end of the day. Imagine the effect it has on the sensory-sensitive systems of the child with autism, especially those with hyper-acute senses. They enter the world with a set of physical challenges that severely impair their ability to tolerate life, let alone within conventional environments. (Grandin 2008, p.112)

The reason researchers like Merzenich and others keep quiet about their findings is because of the possibility of overreaction – such as placing children into overprotective environments. Soundless rooms are not the solution. There should be a clear distinction between the quality of the sensory environment and sensory deprivation.

Since all the senses appear to be involved in difficulties of sensory processing, this indicates some underlying cortical pathology (Baruth *et al.* In press). Research shows that autism is clearly associated with neuropathology of cortical inhibitory interneurons (Casanova 2006; Casanova *et al.* 2002a, b; Levitt 2005) and an imbalance of cortical excitation and inhibition (Rubenstein and Merzenich 2003). Recently there has been active research of the basic units of neocortical function, known as minicolumns (Mountcastle 1997; Silberberg et al. 2002). Minicolumns are defined as the smallest units of the brain capable of processing information; they are vertical columns of functionally related glutamatergic and gamma-aminobutyric acid (GABA)ergic neurons that together process thalamic input. GABAergic local circuit neurons are thought to participate in controlling the functional integrity of minicolumns and providing lateral inhibition of activity from bordering minicolumns (Casanova and Switala 2005; Lund, Angelucci and Bressloff 2003; Peters and Sethares 1997; Raghanti et al. 2010). Comparative studies of minicolumns in the brains of non-autistic and autistic individuals have revealed that in the non-autistic neocortex information is transmitted through the core of the minicolumn and is prevented from activating neighbouring units by surrounding inhibitory fibres. Minicolumns in autism, however, are smaller, more numerous and have abnormal structure (Casanova et al. 2002a), so stimuli are no longer contained within them but rather overflow to adjacent units thus creating an amplifier effect. Inhibitory fibres just do not cope with this flow (Casanova 2006). To illustrate the phenomenon, Casanova (2006) compares inhibitory fibres with a shower curtain. When working properly and fully protecting the bathtub, the shower curtain prevents water from spilling to the floor. In autism, 'water is all over the floor'. Processes that increase the numerical or functional balance of excitatory versus inhibitory cells or effects can lead to a hyper-excitable state. Tito describes the subjective experience of this:

> Panic took over my eyes, blinding them shut. It took over my ears, deafening me with the sound of scream, which was my own… My existence became the sound of that scream… My body and my surroundings were dissolved in the sound generated by my scream. Once it took control, I knew no one had any power to stop it. I had no power to stop it either. (Mukhopadhyay 2008, p.41)

Thus, Gestalt perception (inability to or difficulty with filtering incoming sensory information) and the inability to stop experiencing sensations make autistic individuals hypersensitive and vulnerable to sensory overload. This brings us to the research of Henry and Kamila Markram and their colleague Tania Rinaldi (Markram, Rinaldi and Markram 2007) who have investigated an animal model of autism, that is, a VPA rat model.[1] The investigation has shown that neuroanatomical changes and behavioural traits in the brains of both VPA rats and autistic humans were similar. One of the most replicated findings in the neurology of autism is increased brain volume which is characterized by cerebral overgrowth in very young children and diminished growth rates in later childhood (Courchesne 2002, 2004). Human autopsy studies suggest that part of the extra volume consists of minicolumns in the cerebral cortex (Casanova 2004). The Markrams have studied minicolumns in VPA rats and discovered striking changes similar to those in autistic brains in humans. Using a technique for recording directly from neurons they found that these circuits were hyperconnected: each minicolumn neuron in a VPA rat has up to 50 per cent more connections than normal. This hyperconnectivity causes the neurons to be hyper-reactive, firing more readily when stimulated. The circuits are also hyperplastic, so they form connections with other neurons more readily than normal.

These researchers have put forward a hypothesis for autism which they call 'the intense world syndrome'. According to their hypothesis, *all* features of autism (social interaction impairments, communication and language problems, cognitive functioning, repetitive behaviours, and so forth) are rooted in the sensory overload experienced by individuals with autism. Autistic people perceive, feel and remember too much. Faced with a bombarding, confusing, baffling and often painful environment, autistic infants withdraw into their own world by shutting down their sensory systems. This brings unfavourable consequences for their social and linguistic development. Repetitive behaviours such as rocking the body, flapping hands and head-banging are seen as an attempt to bring order and predictability to their environment.[2] These Swiss researchers have provided strong neurological evidence of the presence of overload in individuals with autism. Contrary to most neurological studies that describe underconnectivity, hypoactivity or deficits of connectivity in autistic brains,[3] the Markrams' research has established that the autistic brain is, in fact, overperforming. The Markrams and Rinaldi (Markram *et al.* 2007) interpret the result of reported underconnectivity and deficits in connection as follows: since highly reactive and autonomous microcircuits may be difficult to activate in a coherent manner with normal stimuli and tasks, they may be hypoactive, but hyper-reactive to a highly selected set of stimuli. Thus, cerebellar responses can be reduced, normal and increased depending on the task. They cite reduced activation reported by other researchers in attention tasks (Allen and Courchesne 2003), in speech recognition and generation (Muller *et al.* 1999), but normal to increased activation during motor tasks (Allen and Courchesne 2003; Allen, Muller and Courchesne 2004).

Hyper-reactivity and hyperplasticity mean that minicolumns have a higher than normal capacity for processing information. Excessive processing of the sensory input in the microcircuits leads, in turn, to exaggerated perception, producing extremely intense images, sounds, smells and so on (Markram *et al.* 2007). This sensory overload, combined with inability to filter information (Gestalt perception; see Bogdashina 2003) causes autistic children to withdraw and miss the opportunity to develop shared conceptual understanding of the world. The Markrams and Rinaldi (Markram *et al.* 2007) show how excessive neuronal processing lead to hyper-perception, hyper-attention and hyper-memory. In this view, ASDs are disorders of hyperfunctionality as opposed to disorders of hypofunctionality, as is often assumed.

> My mind…has been stretched and stretching since the moment of my conception. My capacity for learning, storing, accessing and utilizing information and idea seems infinite beyond belief. I have even referred to myself as 'a human

sponge' and compared my brain to a finely organized computer. (Kochmeister 1995, p.10)

Excessive neuronal processing may make the world painfully intense when the neocortex is affected and even aversive when the amygdala is affected (Markram *et al.* 2007).

Thus, the 'intense world syndrome' interpretation of autism suggests that the autistic person may perceive his or her surroundings as overwhelmingly intense (due to hyper-reactivity of primary sensory areas) and aversive and highly stressful (due to a hyper-reactive amygdala, which makes quick and powerful fear associations with usually neutral stimuli). Impaired social interactions and withdrawal are thus seen as the consequences and not the core features of autism. For example:

> If you were being FOREVER forced (at times none too patiently) to do upsetting functions or at times acutely painful ones, just because everybody else does it with no discomfort, AND expects you to be the same; would that make you outgoing, and a party personality? *Or*, would you turn away from your tormentors, acting as if you were uncomfortable or afraid or possibly frustrated with them? (Morris 1999)[4]

It is important to add, however, that an 'autistic state' is not only about the autistic individual's 'intense world' (and their difficulty coping with it). It is also about their different interpretation of the world around them because of their lack of shared experiences, and their consequent development of different cognitive and linguistic functions. It would be a more useful comparison to call this 'intensely perceived world' a 'parallel world' (differently perceived) as it inevitably would be interpreted, understood and acted on differently (Bogdashina 2003, 2006).

Unlike 'normal' people, at the stage of sensation many autistic individuals perceive everything without filtration and selection and experience the difficulty of distinguishing between foreground and background sensory stimuli. This results in a paradoxical phenomenon: sensory information is received in infinite detail and holistically at the same time, known as 'Gestalt perception' – perception of the whole scene as a single entity with all the details perceived (not processed!) simultaneously (Bogdashina 2003, 2004, 2005).

> Sensory information seems to come to the autistic individual in infinite detail and holistically, that is all at once. It is often hard for the autistic person to integrate what they are experiencing into separate and unique entities. Also, they are very sensitive to many stimuli that most people ignore... Since their parents are usually not autistic, they are often of little help to the autistic child in sorting out sensory information and making sense of their world. This is the first step that begins the loneliness that most autistic people feel for much of their life. (Joan and Rich 1999)

Depending on their individual sensory perceptual profile autistic people may experience Gestalt perception in any sensory modality. A person who experiences visual gestalt has great difficulty in separating a single detail of the scene from the whole picture (without this detail, the whole scene would look different). People with auditory Gestalt perception seem to pick up all the sounds with equal intensity and cannot isolate, for example, the words of the person they are talking to from other noises in the room and so on. If we add their ability to detect stimuli 'normal' people are unaware of, the picture becomes even more complicated:

> The distant noises on the main road that ran about sixty metres from our house were always present. They sloshed against the day-to-day sounds of my own home in sort of wave-on-the-shore effect. I could feel the sensation of cars and a heavy-laden truck pass, and also feel my own physical response to the noises that the vehicle made from its tyres, its engine and the wind of its passing. That wind could suddenly drown out a nearer sound, but not consistently. (Blackman 2001, p.35)

Gestalt perception can account for both strengths and weaknesses in autistic people's perception. On the one hand, this amount of unselected information cannot be processed simultaneously and may lead to sensory information overload, fragmented perception, delayed processing, distortions, mono-processing, peripheral perception and so forth.[5]

Donna Williams describes how this feels from the inside:

> Without developing the capacity to filter out a large amount of incoming sensory information, our conscious minds would be confused and overwhelmed, our perception fragmented, our senses overloaded and perhaps heightened as the mind focused even more intensely on what was coming in in a futile attempt to combat the confusion. Emotions, unprocessed, undefined and all muddled, may terrify us. People, as a major source of ever-changing sensory input may become a source of threatening overload we'd learn to seek to avoid. (Williams 1998, p.82)

No one with 'normal' perception could guess that their eyes, for example, pick up very different signals from light, shade, colour and movement than autistic individuals do. Lucy Blackman describes her experience of the discrepancy between her own and her school teacher's perception of a face, for example:

> The faces my teachers trained me to draw had nothing to do with what I conceptualised as a face. I had no idea why the face I was expected to draw had a circle as its starting-point and two smaller circles in the top half, with a horizontal line or curve below. Though I learnt to label these strange shapes as 'faces', I knew that faces were not like that. Faces consisted of shadows. A pair of small circular shadows inside the eye. More important was the pair of long mouth-to-inner-eye shadows which ran along the nose. When not moving in speech, laughter or fury, the mouth was a comfortable slit-shaped shadow, not much wider than the base of the protuberance above. The rest of the space – eyeballs, forehead,

cheeks, eyebrows, lips, chin – was not shadowed enough to catch my visual processing system... The faces of my private universe were uncontoured, without the slants and slopes and little curves which accompany eye, ear and mouth movements. (Blackman 2001, p.27)

The routines of life and day-to-day connections which most people take for granted may be painfully overwhelming, non-existent or just confusing (Lawson 1998). However, it is not only non-autistic people who cannot imagine that it is possible to perceive the same environment differently; the same is true for individuals with autism. They are often unaware that they perceive the world differently from the other 99 per cent of the population, because they have nothing to compare their perception with (Morris 1999). Wendy Lawson had the following experience:

I think I knew I was different, but I didn't know why. My world was a rich one, full of colour and music that seemed to splash over and around me wherever I walked. I thought everyone saw things the same way I did, but my behaviour seemed to make people angry or cause them to distance themselves from me. (Lawson 1998, p.40)

The first realization of their difficulties usually comes for autistic individuals in the late teens or even later (Lawson 2001; Willey 1999). It may come as a kind of revelation, as well as a blessed relief, when they learn that their sensory problems are not the result of their weakness or lack of character. However, as people around them are often unaware of their different perception, they do not make any effort to accommodate and adjust to these differences. A good mental exercise to get an idea of what it might be like is provided by Spicer:

Suppose you are colour-blind, and cannot distinguish between red and green. You are in a room with other people, all of whom have normal vision. No one – even you – knows that you are colour-blind. Everyone is handed a list of instructions.

They are printed in red against a green background. Everyone except you knows exactly what to do. They cannot understand why you just sit there. The paper looks blank to you, and you cannot understand how the others know what to do. Think of how you would feel, especially if the others stared at you, or whispered, or laughed. (Spicer 1998)

Notes

1. The VPA rat model of autism is based on case studies of children whose mothers were prescribed the anticonvulsant and mood-stabilizing drug valproic acid (VPA). A high proportion of these children (about 10%) developed some form of autism.

2. For a psychological and cognitive theory of sensory perceptual issues at the root of autism see Bogdashina 2003, 2004, 2005.

3. For example, in a short review article on the pathophysiology of autism (Deeley 2009) there are about 30 references to hypoactivation, reduced connectivity, underconnectivity, deficits of connectivity and so on in the brains of autistic individuals, and only one reference to local overconnectivity, in an article by Courchesne and Pierce (2005).

4. Bob Morris (1999) develops his argument further, showing that attempted use of different sensory perceptual mechanisms by a baby *without* any help from a perceptive carer to sort out and deal with these differences (both problems and abilities) may aggravate the condition. The earlier the carer understands the differences and accommodates the person via the appropriate intervention, the more likely the individual will become fully functional, but *significantly different (in talents and thinking)*.

5. See detailed analysis in Bogdashina 2003, 2004, 2005.

SENSORY PERCEPTUAL DEVELOPMENT 5

We are not born with knowledge and ready-made strategies for perceiving and interpreting the complexities of environmental stimuli. Infants acquire information about the world and constantly check the validity of that information. This process defines perception: extracting information from stimulation (Gibson 1969) and shaping it into meaningful (for the culture the baby is born into) units. Our earliest experiences are sensory-based. Babies are flooded with sensations through all their sensory channels and actively create the perceptual world with all its categories through their experiences, memories and cognitive processes. For babies, even their body does not exist as a whole, rather as 'separate organs such as hands, mouth, arms and belly' and they know 'nothing of the various parts being related together' (Tustin 1974, p.60). Gradually babies learn to 'feel self' and control their body parts to produce meaningful movements. Vision or hearing means the ability to receive sights or sounds. However, we have to learn how to see and hear with meaning. We develop our visual and auditory processing skills and achieve comprehension through interaction with the environment. Babies are learning how to discriminate different stimuli from a chaos of sounds, shapes, patterns, movements, and in the first months of their lives infants achieve the ability to make fine discrimination between the slightest variations in colour, form, sound and so on. They actually *learn* how to use their sensory organs and connect sensory images with meaning.[1] With development and maturation, and by interacting with the environment, 'normal' infants learn to sort out incoming information and stop sensory flooding (Williams 2003a). Sensory experiences become linked with one another and become patterned. These are so-called non-verbal (or pre-verbal) ways of knowing about the self and environment. They may be seen as 'sensory abstractions' ('non-verbal thoughts') which are still not sufficiently understood or appreciated. According to Winnicott (1960, 1963) this is the basis of the 'true self' experience, which derives directly from the world-as-experienced and has its origins in the earliest sensations.

'Sensory knowing' starts with recognition of patterns and they are less accessible to conscious, verbal, rational thought (Charles 1999; Stern 1994). Memories of very early experiences (before the appearance of verbal language) become stored and expressed as sensations rather than in highly elaborate form (Innes-Smith 1987). These early experiences are remembered and yet not easily accessible. Affective memories appear to exist prior to, and to some extent separate from, cognitive memories; they influence secondary processes whether or not this influence becomes conscious (Bucci 1997; Krystal 1988). Barsalou (1999) argues that cognition, in fact, is inherently perceptual, sharing systems with perception at both the cognitive and neural levels. This type of attunement serves as the basis of amodal experiences in which incoming information is translated from one sensory modality into another while maintaining the underlying pattern (Stern 1985). Very early in life, infants focus their attention selectively on different aspects of experience, integrate them in memory, and construct simulators to represent objects and events (Cohen 1991; Jones and Smith 1993; Mandler 1992). By the time infants are ready for language, they have a huge amount of knowledge shared with their carers in place to support its acquisition (Barsalou 1999). Matte-Blanco (1975) suggests that 'the sensation is, in itself, a primary experience' (p.101), which is impossible to describe verbally.

In 'normal' development, sensory experience becomes transformed into verbal thought, and verbal thought becomes realized through this primary experience, in their ongoing interplay as alternately container and contained (Bion 1963). However, the tendency to conceptualize development in terms of linear progression is wrong and often brings the confusion between primary process as a non-verbal mode of thinking versus primary process as a developmentally prior and presumably less developed or less complex mode of thinking (Charles 2001). The capacity to form abstractions enables us to move beyond what is literally 'sensed' to what is understood or known at a verbal level. However, at times it is the capacity to enact what has eluded verbal understanding that brings us closer to that very real understanding (Kumin 1996). Charles (2001) admits that even in the psychoanalytic literature with its deep appreciation for the complexity and subtlety of unconscious processes, we still find a tendency to refer to pre-verbal experiences as developmentally prior to or more primitive than conscious thought. They might be more usefully conceptualized as 'primary' modes of experience because, although verbal and rational ways of knowing become more dominant over time, they do not take the place of, nor are they necessarily more complex than, more implicit ways of knowing (Charles 2001). The problem results from our difficulty in conceptualizing multi-dimensional processes (Johnson-Laird 1989) which can be linked to unconscious processes operating 'in a space of a higher number of dimensions than that of our perceptions and conscious thinking' (Matte-Blanco 1988, p.91). Although verbal capacities develop from the non-verbal ones, the two ways of knowing do not represent a continuum and they are not in opposition with one another; they develop alongside each other as two interactive systems, according to different sets of rules (Matte-Blanco 1975).

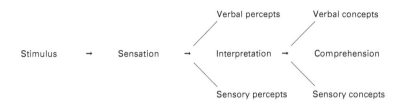

In terms of Bergson's philosophy, verbal and non-verbal capacities are:

> two profoundly different ways of knowing a thing. The first implies that we move round the object; the second, that we enter into it. The first depends on the point of view at which we are placed and on the symbols by which we express ourselves. The second neither depends on the point of view nor relies on any symbol. (Bergson 1912/1999, p.21)

Here we may distinguish two types of consciousness: thought consciousness and sensory consciousness – where the central issue is not thinking but feeling – 'of being alive and living in the presence of sensation' (Humphrey 2002, p.368).[2]

Subconscious, unconscious and preconscious cognitive processes

The way we perceive the world affects the way we store and utilize information, especially memory and thinking. The conscious mind is not the only way of receiving information about the world. What is more, different neural mechanisms are responsible for producing conscious and unconscious processing (Farah and Feinberg 1997; Gazzaniga 1988). Research on blindsight has established that unconscious processing can occur in the absence of conscious realization of visual images (Cowey and Stoerig 1991; Weiskrantz 1996; Weiskrantz et al. 1974). For example, the patient whose right visual cortex was damaged resulting in his being blind on the left side was asked to point to the object displayed at his left. Though being consciously blind (and not seeing the object) the patient could point accurately at it. Director of the Center for Brain and Cognition at the University of California, San Diego (UCSD), Vilyanur S. Ramachandran (2003) provides an explanation of this phenomenon: There are two major visual pathways in the brain – the old (evolutionarily ancient) visual pathway (the superior colliculus) in the brain stem, and the new pathway (the visual cortex) in the back of the brain. The new pathway is responsible for what we usually think of as vision – recognizing objects consciously; the old pathway, on the other hand, is involved in locating objects in the visual field. The patient with the damaged visual cortex (the new pathway) is consciously blind; however, his old pathway (the superior colliculus) works as a back-up. So even though the message from the eyes and optic nerves does not reach the visual cortex (because it is damaged), it takes a parallel route to the superior colliculus which allows the person to locate (unconsciously) the object in space. The message then gets relayed to higher brain centres in the parietal lobes that guide the hand movement accurately to point at the object the person does not see consciously. This explanation suggests that only the new pathway is conscious – events in the old pathway, going through the colliculus and guiding the hand movement, can occur without the person being consciously aware of them (Ramachandran 2003).[3]

Research on preconscious processing shows that conscious states may not accompany unconscious processing, and if they do, they follow it (Velmans 1991). Similarly, conscious awareness follows unconscious processing sensations and initiating actions (Dennett and Kinsbourne 1992). Research on skill acquisition indicates that conscious awareness fades as soon as automaticity develops, leaving unconscious mechanisms largely in control (Shiffrin 1988).[4]

By distinguishing unconscious perceptual processing from conscious perceptual experience we may view those individuals who are mostly verbal thinkers and experience little or no imagery as people whose unconscious perceptual processing underlies cognition with little conscious awareness. If human knowledge is inherently perceptual, there is no a priori reason why it must be represented consciously (Barsalou 1999). Even without conscious awareness we still continue to experience events and accumulate information. For example, both phenomena (change blindness and inattentional blindness) suggest that unattended stimuli are 'seen' (unconsciously or implicitly) at early levels of processing, but not registered consciously. Thus, in autism, even unattended, the information is absorbed (Gestalt) and will be processed later. For example, one time Tito and his mother visited their friends. Tito spent his time there preoccupied by sniffing the pages of a glossy magazine while missing any other objects and furniture in the house. It was on his way home, far from that real room, when he began actually to 'see' that room with all the furniture, curtains, piano and personal things in front of his eyes, recalling the smell of individual items in vivid detail (Mukhopadhyay 2008).

We are limited in our ability to process information consciously. However, subconsciously and/or preconsciously it is possible to take in an infinite amount of unprocessed information which is literal and objective and is received indirectly, without conscious interpretation. The storing capacity is also unlimited. However, the access and retrieval of this information is difficult: it can be triggered but not accessed voluntarily (Williams 1998):

> The conscious mind is limited in its learning. It is slow and plodding and limited in the storage of information. On the other hand, the preconscious state in the absence of mind is indiscriminate. It doesn't filter incoming information in terms of personal or relative significance and takes in a wider scope of information than the conscious mind can. It takes it in at lightning speed and because it doesn't need to interpret that information it purely accumulates it and maps it... [T]he storage capacity of the preconscious state is, by comparison to the conscious mind, virtually infinite. The retrieval system, too, is different. Retrieval of preconsciously accumulated

uninterpreted information is not through conscious voluntary attempts at accessing but through automatic triggering – as in a suggestive post-hypnotic state. (Williams 1998, p.45)

Donna Williams' writing (1999a, 1998) describes the process of receiving knowledge from subconscious to preconscious to conscious, where the subconscious mind is a storeroom containing uninterpreted information that is still accumulated within preconsciousness where it can be processed later, removed from its context. When it is triggered and is perceived consciously after it has been expressed it is like 'listening in on oneself' (Williams 1998).

Some autistic people use the preconscious system to take in information. They use their senses peripherally. It allows them to take in a great amount of information though they themselves are 'absent' from the process. That is, they are not aware of what information they have accumulated, though it may be triggered from the outside. They surprise not only those around them but often themselves as well with their knowledge we have never thought they have. It is sort of 'unknown knowing' (Williams 1996).

By distinguishing between preconscious and subconscious perceptual processing, we can distinguish between different types of intelligence – conscious and preconscious, and subconscious, the latter with little conscious awareness ('unknown knowing'). Armstrong-Buck describes a Whiteheadian analytic approach to these issues. Whitehead believed that most experience is not conscious, that language, though crucial to thought, is not essential to it, and that feeling is the fundamental mode of disclosure of the world. According to Whitehead, thought is not originally verbal or even gestural, though the 'excitation' which is a thought does require expression of some sort (cited in Armstrong-Buck 1989). Propositions are non-linguistic entities and are usually entertained not only without language but without consciousness. Propositions are quasi-physical, in that they are 'lures for feeling' at the unconscious physical level. Armstrong-Buck described these non-verbal propositions in animal research as 'natural concepts' understood observationally as a consistent response to a category of perceived objects or events. 'Natural concepts are based on perceptual abstraction and are abstract to varying degrees' (Armstrong-Buck 1989, p.4).

Perceptual symbol systems can implement cognitive functions naturally and powerfully (Barsalou 1999). It is traditional for perceptually based systems to be seen as recording systems which do not interpret what each part of a recording contains, whereas a conceptual system interprets the entities in a recording. Barsalou (1999) has put forward a perceptual theory of knowledge that demonstrates that a perceptual system is *not* restricted to a recording system but constitutes a fully functional conceptual system. This approach changes how we think about basic cognitive processes, including categorization, concept formation, attention, memory, language, problem solving, decision making, skill, reasoning and formal symbol representation (Barsalou 1999).

Processes of generalization and abstraction are often seen as distinguishing features of verbal rather than non-verbal domains. The concrete is the basis for any understanding, whereas abstraction has the effect, by removing the concrete and particular, of eliminating aspects that obscure the relationship of one element to another (Bion 1963). However, abstraction is not necessarily always a function of verbal meanings, but rather pertains to semantic relations that may or may not be verbal in form (Johnson-Laird 1989). Charles (2001) analyses the interaction between these two levels of experience and finds that it is not so different from physiological processes that go on without our awareness, and yet can be affected by both conscious and unconscious thoughts. Donna Williams provides a useful description of how interpretation and impression inter-connect for her:

> [In autism] an experience may be stored without interpretation, purely on the level of impression…it may be a sensory mapping of an experience linked to a sensation. Still there is no differentiation as to whether the experience is wanted

or not and yet that stored connection may be triggered. That thought may, itself, drive the involuntary response of reaching for or pushing away or a replay of the physical responses that occurred with the original experience.

Without interpretation, there is still experience. Without interpretation there is still sensation and emotion. Without interpretation there is a form of involuntary thought, expression and action. (Williams 1998, p.96)

It is important to understand and communicate semantic relations that had been unknown in the verbal domain. A lack of appreciation of the non-verbal domains leaves our thinking insubstantial and trivialized, cut off from its roots.

Life at either extreme obviously has its drawbacks, but our culture seems to elevate the verbal channels to a point where meaning is diminished... An appreciation of the intertwining and interweaving of the verbal and non-verbal domains of experience may help us to value each without pathologizing either. (Charles 2001)

Charles Darwin argued that mental abilities are continuous from one animal species to the next, and differences in mental abilities are not differences in *kind* but differences in *degree* along a continuum. Henry Bergson disagreed with this view. In his book *Creative Evolution* (1911/1944), Bergson distinguishes between three very marked tendencies – torpor, instinct and intelligence – which, he insists, are not three successive stages in the linear development of one tendency, but three diverging directions of development, which split up as it went on its way. According to Bergson, instinct and intelligence are the two important terminal points in evolution, and not two stages of which one is higher than the other – they are at the end of two different routes. Bergson gives an example to show the contrast between instinct and intelligence: a cat knows how to nurture her new-born kittens; a human mother has to be taught how to raise her children or observe how others do it. A cat performs her simple duties by instinct; a human mother has to use her intelligence to perform hers. In humans, intellect is seen at its best; in ants and bees and such creatures, instinct is the sole guide of a highly organized life. The value of each is relative. Thus, while instinct is far more perfect and complete in its insight, it is confined within narrow limits. Intelligence, on the other hand, while far less perfect in accomplishing its work and less complete in its insight, is not limited in such a way. While intellect is external, looking on reality as different from life, instinct is an inner sympathy with reality; it is deeper than any intellectual bond which binds the conscious creature to reality, because it is a vital bond (Bergson 1911/1944). Bergson's doctrine of intuition can be summarized as follows:

> Instinct is sympathy... [I]ntelligence and instinct are turned in opposite directions, the former toward inert matter, the latter toward life. Intelligence, by means of science...goes all round life, taking from outside the greatest possible number of views of it, drawing in into itself instead of entering it. But it is to the very inwardness of life that *intuition* leads us – by intuition I mean instinct that has become disinterested, self-conscious, capable of reflecting upon its object and of enlarging it indefinitely. (Bergson 1911/1944, p.194)

> By intuition is meant the kind of *intellectual sympathy* by which one places oneself within an object in order to coincide with what is unique in it and consequently inexpressible. Analysis, on the contrary, is the operation which reduces the object to elements already known, that is, to elements common to it and other objects. To analyse, therefore, is to express a thing as a function of something other than itself. All analysis is thus a translation, a development into symbols, a representation taken from successive points of view from which we are studying and others which we believe we know already... Analysis multiplies without the end the number of points of view in order to complete its always incomplete representation, and ceaselessly varies its symbols that it may

perfect the always imperfect translation… But intuition…is a simple act. It is an act directly opposed to analysis, for it is a viewing in totality, as an absolute; it is a synthesis, not analysis, not an intellectual act, for it is an immediate, emotional synthesis. (Bergson 1912/1999, pp.23–24)

Similar ideas are expressed by Belenky *et al.* (1986) who distinguish between *understanding*, predicated on personal acquaintance with the object, involving 'intimacy and equality between self and other' versus *knowledge*, implying 'separation from the subject and mastery over it' (p.101). These are reflections of two ways of knowing: non-verbal versus verbal. Carl Jung (1923) distinguished four basic psychic (mental) functions: two rational – thinking and feeling; and two irrational – sensing and intuition. Whorf (1956) comments that thinking, as defined by Jung, contains a large linguistic element, while feeling is mainly non-linguistic, though it may use language in a different way from thinking. By contrast, sensing and intuition may be termed non-linguistic.

Bergson's 'intellectual sympathy' can be seen in a phenomenon experienced by some autistic people – 'losing oneself' in the stimuli to the extent that one can become 'resonant' with them. These terms were introduced by Donna Williams to define a state when one 'loses oneself in' or 'resonates with' something else: 'I would resonate with the sensory nature of object with such an absolute purity and loss of self that it was like an overwhelming passion into which you merge and become part of beauty itself' (Williams 1998, p.15).

In her books, Donna Williams gives many examples of what it feels like to resonate with surroundings, too. This is one of them:

> When I was about ten years old I used to have a certain colour billiard ball – a pink one. I used to spend around an hour with it before I could reach the point of resonance with it where I would merge with the colour. To anyone else this would have looked like some 'psychotic' but if they'd known the physical alteration felt in that moment of becoming one with a colour some people would perhaps see it as far less

crazy than other ways many people may have spent an hour of their lives at the same age. (Williams 1998, p.22)

Some autistic individuals seem to be able to surpass the most skilled 'normal' people in resonating with their surroundings. Those who experience this condition can be 'in resonance' with colours, sounds, objects, places, plants, animals, people. For example:

I could resonate with the cat and spent hours lying in front of it, making no physical contact with it. I could resonate with the tree in the park and feel myself merge with its size, its stability, its calm and its flow. (Williams 1998, p.44)

When 'in resonance' with people, autistic individuals can sense ('see', 'hear', etc.) the thoughts, emotions, pain and so forth of other people, for example:

When I was younger I heard a lot of noises in my head, spoken things and unspoken things. Tell me you can hear people think. I wish I didn't. If there is a medication that will kill people's thoughts I'd like to try it. (Walker and Cantello 1994)

I…remember responding to people's calls by coming into the room, sometimes answering their request by going and getting what they'd wanted. People had seemed surprised at these behaviours because they hadn't spoken the requests. It didn't occur to me that I hadn't been verbally called or asked or thought that I was busy with things of my own at the time. (Williams 1998, p.27)

The person can merge with different sensory stimuli as if the person becomes the stimulus itself. These are very real experiences. For example, Donna Williams describes how she could 'feel' colours:

[The] street lights were yellow with a hint of pink but in a buzz state they were an intoxicating iridescent-like pink-yellow. My mind dived deeper and deeper into the colour, trying to feel its nature and become it as I progressively lost sense of self in its overwhelming presence. Each of the colours resonated different feelings within me and it was like they played me as a chord, where other colours played one note at a time. (Williams 1999a, p.19)

Wendy Lawson describes her experience when the colours and fragrance were so vibrant to her senses that she could 'feel' them. While watching some shiny things she felt a sense of connection; she felt safe, as if she were part of them. Lawson (1998) writes 'I felt so intoxicating and I felt so alive'. This can be compared with Huxley's experience of fascination or resonance:

The legs…of that chair – how miraculous their tubularity, how supernatural their polished smoothness! I spent several minutes – or was it several centuries? – not merely gazing at those bamboo legs, but actually being them – or rather being myself in them; or, to be still more accurate (for 'I' was not involved in the case, nor in a certain sense were 'they') being my Not-self in the Not-self which was the chair. (Huxley 1954/2004, p.10)

However, there may be side-effects of these experiences when the person loses the sense of self, becoming Not-self, and perceiving and being simultaneously all things around this new-born Not-self (Huxley 1954/2004).

During meditation people can achieve similar experiences:

People think of reality as some sort of guarantee they can rely on. Yet from the earliest age I can remember I found my only dependable security in losing all awareness of the things usually considered real. In doing this, I was able to lose all sense of self. Yet this is the strategy said to be the highest stage of meditation, indulged in to achieve inner peace and tranquillity. Why should it not be interpreted as such for autistic people? (Williams 1999a, p.178)

Donna Williams saw 'Her World' (or 'simply be') as a place of richness and beauty where language was not through words. 'Her World' outside of 'simply be' was a place where the only state of security she could achieve was through non-existence. 'The system of "simply be" was a way to experience the self you normally are deaf, blind, and dead to in the world' (Williams 1999b, p.176). Further, Donna hypothesizes that some autistic individuals had their own worlds but they had either never known the addictive beauty and peace of 'simply be' or else they had lost it too long ago to remember.

The experiences of 'oneness' with the world are comparable to religious feelings:

> [Once, working in a plant]…my religious feelings were renewed… I felt totally at one with the universe as I kept the animals completely calm while the rabbi performed shehita. Operating the equipment there was like being in a Zen meditation state. Time stood still, and I was totally, completely disconnected from reality… It was a feeling of total calmness and peace… The experience had been… strangely hypnotic… I thought about the similarities between the wonderful trancelike feeling I had had while gently holding the cattle in the chute and the spaced-out feeling I had had as a child when concentrating on dribbling sand through my fingers on the beach. During both experiences all other sensation was blocked.
>
> […] Maybe the monks who chant and meditate are kind of autistic. I have observed that there is a great similarity between certain chanting and praying rituals and the rocking of an autistic child. I feel there has to be more to this than just getting high on my endorphins… When the animal remained completely calm I felt an overwhelming feeling of peacefulness, as if God had touched me… As the life force left the animal, I had been completely overwhelmed with feelings I did not know I had. (Grandin 1998, pp.204–205)

There is no deeper experience than the total encapsulation of self within an experience until one is indistinguishable from the experience. It is like knowing 'God'. (Williams 1998, p.58)

Another interesting feature of the state of 'resonance' is when one can sense the surface, texture and density of material without looking at it with physical eyes or touching it with physical hands or tasting it with a physical tongue or tapping it to hear how it sounds, that is, sensing it with non-physical senses (the so-called 'shadow senses' (Williams 1998)):

Before we learned to use our physical-body senses with intention, we were still able to see, hear, feel with 'shadow senses'... one does not need words to shadow-sense the coming of pattern changes before hearing the impending changes voiced through a hole in the face or visually cued. Here one does not need to touch an object to feel its nature; the feeling of the nature is not, at this stage, from a place of body separateness, it is to feel the object *as* the object, from within, without interpretation or mind, using the body not as a tool of sensory exploration or body as self, but as a tool of resonance. (Williams 1998, p.26)

Researchers are catching up with these phenomena (see Rosenblum, Wuestefeld and Saldaña 1993; Rosenblum, Wuestefeld and Anderson 1996). Rosenblum and colleagues conducted experiments in which blind and sighted but blindfolded subjects were asked to walk towards a movable wall placed at different distances from their starting point. The subjects were able to signal when they began to sense the presence of the wall without touching it. Our brains are capable of taking many different sensory inputs and combining them in unusual ways (Ramachandran cited in LaFee 2007). These experiments show that we can hear the silent environment because surroundings not only make sounds we are not consciously aware of, but they also structure them; they give them shape, which people can 'see' without seeing (Rosenblum cited in LaFee 2007).

Donna Williams describes a developmental route from 'shadow' to 'physical senses': 'I moved from sensing through "becoming one" with matter ("resonance") to using touch. Instead of merely "taking on" the things around me in a sort of merging, I now began reaching out physically as separate entities' (Williams 1998, p.55).

An American philosopher of Harvard, William James (1884), hypothesized that in a way a stream of (unlimited) consciousness is reduced and distorted by intellect which frames it into concepts. By its nature, intellect is the fabricator of concepts, and concepts are static; they leave out the flux of things, omitting too much of experience and losing vital contact with life itself. Bergson states that the original form of consciousness was nearer to intuition than to intelligence. With development, man has found intellect more valuable for practical use, yet intuition is still there:

> ...but vague and, above all, discontinuous. It is a lamp almost extinguished which only glimmers now and then for a few moments at most. But it glimmers whenever a vital interest is at stake. On our personality, on our liberty, on the place we occupy in the whole of Nature, on our origin, and perhaps also on our destiny, it throws a light, feeble and vacillating, but which, none the less, pierces the darkness of the night in which the Intellect leaves us. (Bergson 1911/1944, pp.291–292)

However, Bergson insists that intellect and intuition are not opposed to each other:

> How could there be a 'disharmony between our Intuition and our Science, how, especially, could our Science make us renounce our Intuition, if these Intuitions are something like Instinct – an Instinct conscious, refined, spiritualized – and if Instinct is still nearer Life than Intellect and Science? (Bergson 1911, p.43)

Bergson does *not* mean that we must return to the standpoint of an animal, which is instinctive. Intuition, to be fruitful, must interact with intellect. It has the direct insight of instinct, but its range is widened as it blends with intellect. Bergson believes that the whole progress of evolution is towards the creation of a type of being whose intuition will be equal to his intelligence (Gunn 1920). The philosopher claims that everyone has had opportunities to exercise intuition in some degree. In a way, our tendency to disown and disregard our non-verbal or intuitive experiences – our elusive sensory knowings – and always to check and verify them with our 'knowledge' means that 'growing up' is often synonymous with growing away from self (Charles 2001).

What Bergson meant under 'intuition' is very similar to what Donna Williams calls 'sensing' – interpreting and comprehending the world through sensory feelings and sensory-based concepts that, unlike verbal concepts, give a literal (and therefore, more accurate) representation of the environment. Some people have trained themselves in the system of sensing, for instance, great artists, musicians and poets. Their genius is their power to penetrate into reality itself and express it in their work. For many autistic individuals intuition is a natural way to interact with the world.

> [In normal development] one filters information and interprets sensory experience and whilst this builds the capacity to filter information, it also begins to limit how we perceive something external to ourselves. We can no longer take it in exactly as it is. Instead, this earlier mapping of relative and personal significance builds a cognitive net and information is taken in terms of how we conceive of it based upon an accumulated and interpreted bunch of information. (Williams 1998, p.56)

Professor Alan Snyder (1997), who has been investigating the abilities of autistic savants, comes to a similar conclusion – in 'normal' development the human brain acts like a filter, passing into consciousness only an edited and highly conceptualized version of the world. In contrast, autism is the state of delayed acquisition of concepts (Snyder, Bossomaier and Mitchell 2004), and autistic people have access to the 'raw sensory information'. We all possess the same lower-level information, but we cannot voluntarily access it (Snyder and Mitchell 1999).[5] This hypothesis builds on research that newborns, unlike adults, are probably aware of the raw sensory data available at lower levels of neural processing and that they quite possibly have excellent recall of this information. With maturation, there is a strategy to suppress such awareness. The maturing mind becomes increasingly aware only of concepts to the exclusion of the details that comprise these concepts. On the other hand, as Snyder (1996) puts it, an autistic mind is more conscious and hence aware of all the details that lead to alternative representations of the world. Snyder hypothesizes that autism may be considered as a 'retarded acquisition of mental paradigms'. At the low-functioning end of the autism spectrum we may find a lack of paradigms across various domains; and at the high-functioning end and in Asperger syndrome individuals can be deficient in only the most elaborate mindsets, such as are necessary for subtle social interaction (Snyder 1996). It is interesting that, because autistic individuals have fewer mental models (verbal concepts) of the world, they can be more aware of novelty (Hermelin 2001; Pring and Hermelin 2002; Snyder *et al.* 2004). Snyder and colleague believe 'that autistic savants have direct access to "lower" levels of neural information prior to it being integrated into the holistic picture, the ultimate label. All of us possess this same lower-level information, but we cannot normally access it' (Snyder and Mitchell 1999, p.588).

However, there are disadvantages to this 'superability', described below:

- Such a mind would have difficulty in coping with the flood of information and would need routines and structure to make sense of the conventional world, because every detail has to be examined anew each time it is perceived and with equal importance to every other detail.

- There would be lack of (or delay in) development of symbolic systems, such as communication, language and verbal thought (Snyder 1996).

> In a world where the system of sensing has been left behind, few who have moved into the system of interpretation have named the mechanics of the system of sensing. Because of this there is little learned means of putting it easily into words. Even if there were, who would listen when most people no longer have the mental construct to slot in such explanations; their minds are reformatted, the old disks just can't be read in the new computer. (Williams 1998, p.125)

The development of 'symbolic' thinking in autism

Donna Williams (1998) distinguishes between two systems of comprehension – the system of sensing and the system of interpretation. Although we possess both capacities – of 'feeling' the outside world and of comprehending it – all our lives, one of the systems becomes dominant in very early childhood and develops rapidly. In 'normal' development the dominant side of interpretation (and later on, communication and thinking) is a verbal (symbolic) one, whereas in autism we may observe sensory-based thinking or, at least, a later occurrence of the transition of dominance from sensory to verbal (symbolic) plane of comprehension.

> In my case, I remember this transition from the system of sensing into the system of interpretation began to happen not in the first days or weeks of life as usual but at around three years old. It was not until around the age of ten that the system of interpretation (with much begrudgement) eventually came to be relied upon rather than merely put up with or tuned out. Even then, it was taken on, not as a first and primary 'language' but as a secondary one and much later as one of two equal but different 'primary' systems. (Williams 1998, p.79)

Some autistic individuals (especially non-verbal individuals with so called low-functioning autism) maintain a sensory-based system all their lives. Some acquire a system of symbols later in life as a secondary (not dominant) system. Still other autistic individuals move to a verbal plane of interpretation, maintaining perceptual thinking.

> I had not developed any disciplined feedback to myself from babbling and internal language, because I had not developed speech. Nor had I really locked the speech that I heard from others into what my body was experiencing, or what I had experienced internally. I got feedback in my memory mainly from sound, sight, taste and emotion that related to the experience that I was undergoing in the immediate present...
>
> ...[T]he speech I had spontaneously developed from childhood was very impromptu, in the sense that the word popped out in response to my internal challenge, and with no link to my thoughts... To complicate things, I had had the problem that I really did not know what speech was for. (Blackman 2001, pp.163, 279)

Autistic children often have difficulty moving from sensory patterns (literal perception) to understanding and forming concepts. For those who are at the stage of literal perception words have no meanings; they are just sound-patterns and may serve as 'auditory toys' to play with. When a small child, Tito did not realize that words had any meaning. For him, they were patterns of wonderful sounds. When his mother was reciting poems, Tito used to play with words in his mind, creating his own rhymes with sound patterns (Mukhopadhyay 2000). For some with severe sensory processing problems, verbal language may be perceived as no more than noise that has nothing to do with either interaction or interpretation of the environment. Donna Williams describes this as: 'Words were a sensory material. They didn't have a use. They were just there. You could map their strings, their shifts and replay them' (Williams 2005). Williams (2003a) hypothesizes that if you cannot integrate information cohesively, it is hard to form concepts; and if you cannot form concepts, you do not learn to filter out all the sensory information coming in. She defines the underlying cause of sensory flooding as the inability to form concepts quickly enough to bring fragments of information cohesively together as a whole. When information comes in, 'it has no structures to slot into' (p.76). Donna states that it is possible to control perception and manage overload by learning to convert fragments into concepts, into a singular context:

> [In an art gallery] I was buzzing on an array of free-floating forms against a big white background. The forms had different edges and curves, seeming almost to swim among the white. Then Mary Kay remarked, 'Oh, you like the painting of the lion,' and something freaky happened. The shapes stopped being just shapes. The whiteness stopped being a square whiteness. I saw a lion, a lion on a white canvas. I was absolutely shocked, as though she had done magic. It was then that I had my first conversation about the power of labels to trigger the concepts that would cause visual cohesion to happen… It taught me I could control overload in a new way, by looking away, tuning out, and struggling for an umbrella term, a folder, for a fragmented experience. (Williams 2003a, pp.77–8)

These differences in conceptualization of sensory information do not mean that autistic individuals remain stuck at the early stage of development. They do develop but via different routes. They develop different concepts and interpretations of what is going on around them, creating what Tito calls 'mental maps', or mental pictures he created and which he expected to encounter in similar situations. Every experience was seen as a natural phenomenon and if it went against the 'rules' Tito had established, he became anxious and did not know how to proceed, for example:

> if I saw a bird on a tree, and, at that very moment, I saw someone walking across the street in front of our gate, I concluded that every time a bird sits on a tree, someone needs to walk across the street. What if they did not happen together? Well, I would panic and get so anxious that I would scream. (Mukhopadhyay 2008, p.7)

Each and every situation is unique. Even the slightest changes in their environment or routine may confuse and upset people with autism. Autistic children can perform in exactly the same situation with exactly the same prompts, but fail to apply the skill if anything in the routine or prompt has been changed.

The process of concept acquisition may be very slow and needs a lot of practice. They learn to move from specific perceptual images to generalized concepts:

> To learn a concept of *dog* or *street*, I had to see many specific dogs or streets before the general concept could be formed. A general concept such as *street* without pictures of many specific streets stored in my memory bank is absolutely meaningless. (Grandin 2008, p.33)

> When I used a word like 'nose', I did not think of it as a representation of the thing that others saw, but as a symbol of my own sensation of being the possessor of the feature. (Blackman 2001, p.61)

Some autistic individuals tend to rely on intuition much more than on what is available at the surface, for example:

> Even once interpretation got progressively on line... I couldn't let go of what I trusted and identified with. I can remember walking down the street even at the age of six and sensing something which was about to happen but then attempting to read (interpret) the situation. I remember, at that time, that I turned from sensing and went with the odds of what I'd interpreted and that it hadn't worked out.

What I'd sensed had been right. I recall cursing myself for not trusting in sensing and attempting to use interpretation. (Williams 1998, p.33)

It is very important to remember that sensory perceptual differences are very real for many people with autism. We all live in the same physical world but for many autistic individuals it looks, sounds, smells, and so on, different. They develop their own concepts to understand it. For example, at one of the sessions a researcher read a story for Tito (to assess his comprehension); however, instead of the story Tito heard the researcher's voice and saw it as long green strings vibrating with different amplitudes and producing a beautiful yellow and green effect around the researcher's mouth. When asked what the story was about, Tito was honest about his experience of the situation and wrote about the beauty of the colour green, when yellow sunshine melts through newly grown leaves. This was the way Tito's perception interpreted it to himself when translating the experience into verbal language (Mukhopadhyay 2008).

> This personal-world reality and the world-as-processed-by-the-eyes are continually confused. From the comments around me, I gather that this is not a problem for the person whose visual field is fine-tuned to the space and speed common to most humans: but to me, and I think to others like me, it is a source of constant misunderstanding. I was an adult before I could explain to anyone the dreadful instability of a scene that could sparkle one minute, and simultaneously have some components in a pastel haze. I would have done so sooner if I had realised that human sight was not like that, and as a result most people positioned each movement of their bodies in a space that was not unstable. (Blackman 2001, p.33)

Being autistic does not mean being inhuman. But it does mean being alien, different. It means that what is normal for other people is not normal for me, and what is normal for me is not normal for other people. In some ways I am terribly ill-equipped to survive in this world, like an extraterrestrial stranded without an orientation manual. (Sinclair 1992, p.302)

Notes

1. Some autistic children may need to be taught how to see (with meaning) using their eyes, how to hear (with meaning) using their ears, how to eat and how to move. Jim Sinclair (1992), a high-functioning person with autism, emphasizes that simple, basic skills such as recognizing people and objects presuppose even simpler, more basic skills such as knowing how to process sounds, that, in turn first require recognizing sounds as things that can be processed, and recognizing processing as a way to extract order from chaos. Autistic individuals may experience problems acquiring these skills. More complex functions such as speech (or any kind of motor behaviour) require the ability to keep track of all the body parts involved, and to coordinate all their movements. Producing any behaviour in response to any perception requires monitoring and coordinating all the inputs and outputs at once, and doing it fast enough to keep up with changing inputs that may call for changing outputs (Sinclair 1992). Some autistic children do not seem to possess these basic, taken for granted by others, abilities.

2. In his book *A History of the Mind: Evolution and the Birth of Consciousness* (1992), Nicholas Humphrey argues that consciousness is essentially a matter of having bodily sensations rather than having higher level thoughts, and proposes a theory of how consciousness may have evolved.

3. When blindsight syndrome was first discovered, it seemed so bizarre that many researchers refused to accept that it existed. But in a sense, we all suffer from blindsight, for instance while driving a car we can be engaged in a conversation with a friend (a conscious experience) and successfully navigate the traffic (without being consciously aware what we are doing and why) (Ramachandran 2003). Similarly, in priming, there is an increased sensitivity to the stimulus that at first was briefly presented but not consciously experienced (see e.g. Marcel 1983). See more on blindsight and its role in the so-called ESP in Chapter 10.

4. So we can distinguish several types or styles of receiving the information which differ in the ways in which perceiving, storing and retrieving information occur:

    *   Conscious mind implies the mental facilities are awake and active.

    *   Preconscious mind contains memories that can be readily made conscious.

- Subconscious mind can be defined as part of the mental field outside the range of attention and therefore outside consciousness.

- Unconscious mind comprises those mental processes whose existence is inferred from their effects.

(Bogdashina 2003)

5. If we all potentially store low level (sensory) information, there might be some artificial means to access it. Snyder and colleagues (Snyder 2001, 2004; Snyder and Thomas 1997; Snyder *et al.* 2003, 2006), for example, have shown that it is possible to induce savant-like skills in 'normal' people by inhibiting the left anterior temporal lobe by transcranial magnetic stimulation (TMS).

HIDDEN AGENDA OF LANGUAGE 6

Huxley hypothesizes that man has developed symbol-systems (languages) to keep awareness reduced and functioning efficient. Every individual is at once the beneficiary and the victim of this linguistic tradition; he takes his concepts for data and his words for actual things (Huxley 1954/2004). 'Normal' perceptions of the outside world are clouded by the verbal notions and concepts in terms of which people do their thinking. In autism language development is qualitatively different. On the one hand, this makes their perception of the world more accurate (and concept-less) and seems to allow better awareness and an extraordinary memory capability. On the other hand, it hinders their functioning in the 'normal' linguistic environment.

> To understand the mind of a child or adult who is completely non-verbal, without oral, sign, or written language, you must leave the world of thinking in words. This can be quite challenging for many people. Our society functions through the spoken word. For the majority of people, words are their 'native language'. It is difficult for them to step outside this very basic way of relating and imagine something else. Some neurotypicals, especially those with stronger creative

sides, can do this. Other neurotypicals struggle immensely in understanding this concept. (Grandin 2008, p.83)

Language is typically defined as a system of symbols (words) and methods (rules), a combination of which is used by a section or group of people and serves as a means of communication and formulating and expressing thoughts. As we discussed earlier, language is one of the systems to reduce awareness and make functioning efficient. The linguistic systems are both beneficial (as language gives an access to the accumulated knowledge of previous generations and other people's experiences) and restrictive (as it reduces awareness by sidelining anything that is not expressed linguistically).

A useful hypothesis

As language is a convention, it is a model of a culture and of its adjustment to the world (Hill 1958). Here we have to turn to a (controversial but useful for our discussion) hypothesis that considers the role of language in cultural development and in the construction of a 'cultural-linguistic world'. It is known as the Sapir-Whorf hypothesis.[1] It starts with the assumption that our view of the world is shaped by the language we learned as a child. Edward Sapir, an outstanding linguist, hypothesized that the 'real' world is to a large extent unconsciously built upon the language habits of the group of people speaking this particular language. The world in which different cultures live are distinct worlds, rather than the same one with different labels attached, as no languages are sufficiently similar to be considered as representing the same social reality (Sapir 1929/1949).

> Human beings do not live in the objective world alone, nor alone in the world of social activity as ordinarily understood, but are very much at the mercy of the particular language which has become the medium of expression for the society. It is quite an illusion to imagine that one adjusts to reality essentially without the use of language and that language

is merely an incidental means of solving specific problems of communication or reflection. The fact of the matter is that the 'real world' is to a large extent unconsciously built up on the language habits of the group... We see and hear and otherwise experience very largely as we do because the language habits of our community predispose certain choices of interpretation. (Sapir 1929/1949, p.162)

Ideas which are similarly compelling are expressed by Wilhelm von Humboldt who states that we live with the objects presented to us by language; it is very hard if not impossible to step out of the 'magic circle' drawn around us by our language (cited in Cassirer 1946). Sapir's thesis was further developed by Benjamin Lee Whorf, a remarkable individual,[2] who defined language as 'a classification and arrangement of the stream of sensory experience which results in a certain world-order, a certain segment of the world that is easily expressible by the type of symbolic means that language employs' (Whorf 1956, p.55).

> Once in a blue moon a man comes along who grasps the relationship between events which have hitherto seemed quite separate, and gives mankind a new dimension of knowledge. Einstein, demonstrating the relativity of space and time, was such a man. In another field and on a less cosmic level, Benjamin Lee Whorf was one... (Chase 1956, p.v)

As evidence for his theory, Whorf studied the language of the Hopi Indians and showed how their views of the world were closely related to the grammatical categories of their language.[3] Whorf introduced the principle of linguistic relativity that reads that 'all observers are not led by the same physical evidence to the same picture of the universe, unless their linguistic backgrounds are similar, or can in some way be calibrated' (Whorf 1956, p.214). For example, our notions of (Newtonian) space and time are thought to be intuitive – we sense or feel that we live and move in space and time. We can go straight to the end of the street, then turn left, climb up the fence and turn right; similarly, we can report what happened yesterday, make plans for today and think about tomorrow. Because we have all these concepts of space and time units (for example, up and down, right and left, square, cube, hour, week, year), we think that it is the way the universe is organized. However, Newtonian space, time and matter are not intuitions. They have come from the culture and language of each particular group (Whorf 1950).

The Sapir-Whorf hypothesis has won both supporters and critics. The main argument to oppose the idea of languages 'shaping' the interpretation of the environment is Chomsky's 'transformational grammar' (1957) – the idea that all languages have common underlying structures ('a universal grammar'). However, as supporters of the Sapir-Whorf hypothesis emphasize, each language arranges different categories in a different way:

> Each language lays down its own boundaries within the amorphous 'thought-mass' and stresses different factors in it in different arrangements, puts the centers of gravity in different places and gives them different emphases. It is like one and the same handful of sand that is formed in different patterns. (Hjelmslev 1961, p.52)

The meaning of any word is closely related to the experiences of the members of each particular culture of the object or event the word refers to. We learn to structure experience and thought as they are structured by a certain social group (Brown 1958), and languages differ in the way they reflect cultural attitudes and experiences. The experience of professional translators and interpreters at the United Nations (UN) supports this view. Edmund S. Glenn has analysed hundreds of UN transcriptions to find differences in concepts reflected in different languages. His analysis showed that while the translation technique was smooth on the surface, the degree of communication between even some Western languages appeared to be nil in some cases. For example, the English speaker says, 'I assume'; the Russian translator interprets it as 'I consider', while the French renders it 'I deduce' (White 1955). Chase (1956) speculates that if there is some difficulty among Western languages, what can we expect from languages outside of the Indo-European group? Languages classify items of experience differently. The class corresponding to one word and one thought (concept) in language A may be regarded by language B as two or more classes corresponding to two or more words and thoughts (concepts) (Whorf 1956). For instance, in the Hopi language studied by Whorf such words (nouns) as 'lightning, wave, flame, meteor, pulsation' are verbs – they describe events of brief duration.

The linguistic relativity hypothesis has received an interesting interpretation in works by Carlos Castaneda (1971, 1972, 1974)[4] who emphasizes that the world we 'see' is no more than one possible description of the reality that is beyond anything we actually know. The same view has been supported by other authors (e.g. Cassirer 1946; Lilly 1972).

The comparison of the Hopi language with English (based on Whorf 1940, 1941, 1950)

> Just as it is possible to have any number of geometries other than the Euclidean which give an equally perfect account of space configurations, so it is possible to have descriptions of the universe, all equally valid, that do not contain our familiar contrasts of time and space. The relativity viewpoint of modern physics is one such view, conceived in mathematical terms, and the Hopi Weltanschauung is another and quite different one, mathematical and linguistic. (Whorf 1950, p.67)

Whorf approached his task with the assumption that it is possible to describe the universe according to the Hopi only by means of approximation and working out new concepts and abstraction to reflect the Hopi view of the universe. In the Hopi view, time disappears and space is altered, and at the same time new concepts enter to describe the world without reference to time and space. The Hopi's metaphysics (which is different from ours) may appear to the Westerners as psychological or even mystical in character. While Western metaphysics imposes on the universe two grand cosmic forms: static three-dimensional space and perpetually flowing time, the Hopi metaphysics contains two grand cosmic forms, which can be described by approximation as *manifested (objective)* and *manifesting, or unmanifest (subjective)*. The objective or manifested represents all that is accessible to the senses, without distinguishing present or past, but excluding everything that we call future. The subjective or manifesting comprises all that we call future (much of which the Hopi regard as predestined) and everything we call mental (including mentality, intellection and emotion), that is, that appears to exist in the mind (in the Hopi's term 'in the heart', not only in the human heart, but in the heart of animals, plants, and so on, in short, in the heart of nature).

Time

The Hopi language does not contain words, grammatical forms or expressions that refer directly to what we call 'time', or to past, present or future; or to enduring or lasting. What we call 'present' is in the realm of subjective in Hopi; it is something that is beginning to emerge into manifestation (comparable to 'going to sleep' or 'starting to write'). It can be approximated to our 'future' that includes a part of our present time; but most of what we call present belongs in Hopi to the objective realm, so similar to our past.

In the Hopi language, it is unclear when 'one' event ends and 'another' begins. It is implicit that everything that ever happened still is, but it is in a different form. As for the present the best word to describe it is 'preparing'. In short, Hopi may be called a timeless language. It does recognize psychological time, which is much like Bergson's 'duration', and not the time used by our physicists. Among the peculiarities of Hopi ('duration') time are that it varies with each observer of the event, does not permit simultaneity, and has zero dimensions, i.e., it cannot be assigned a number greater than one. For example, 'I stayed five days' in Hopi will be 'I left on the fifth day'.

Space

In Hopi, there is no space in the objective sense; it is in the subjective realm. However, it seems to be symbolically related to the vertical dimension, going through the zenith and the underground, as well as to the 'heart' of things (which corresponds to the word 'inner' in the metaphorical sense). From each subjective axis, there extends the objective realm in every physical direction. Its distance includes what we call time in the sense of the temporal relation between events. Things at a distance from the observer do not happen simultaneously: what happens in a distant village can only be known objectively when events are 'past', and the more distant, the more 'past'.

Whorf concludes that concepts of 'time' and 'space' are not given in the same form by experience to all men but depend on the nature of languages through which they have developed. Our 'time' differs considerably from Hopi 'duration'. Though there is no striking difference between our concept of 'space' and the Hopi concept (we see things in the same space forms as the Hopi), still 'space' as sensed by the Hopi would be comparatively 'pure', free from such extraneous notions as intensity, tendency, and so on.[5]

'Primitive' languages

Having studied the languages of the American Indians (which were often referred to as 'primitive'),[6] Whorf discovered a seeming paradox – a 'primitive' language is much better equipped than a 'sophisticated and well-developed' one to deal with physical science. Some languages, Whorf believes, are closer to reality; their concepts are a more accurate reflection of the world we know. For example, when we look at a surface in everchanging undulating motions, we say 'see that wave', but a wave cannot exist by itself. Some languages do not have a word for 'a wave'; they are closer to reality in this respect. Hopi say *walalata*, 'plural waving occurs' (Whorf 1956). Another example of more accurate (scientific) reflection of reality is in verbs without subjects that give a better understanding of certain aspects, for example, 'flash (occurred)'.

> We are constantly reading into nature fictional entities, simply because our verbs must have substantives in front of them. We have to say 'It flashed' or 'A light flashed', setting up an actor, 'it' or 'light', to perform what we call an action, 'to flash'. Yet the flashing and the light are one and the same! The Hopi language reports the flash with a simple verb, *rehpi*: 'flash (occurred)'... Undoubtedly modern science, strongly reflecting western Indo-European tongues, often does as we all do, sees actions and forces where it sometimes might be better to see states. (Whorf 1956, pp.243–244)

> According to the conceptions of modern physics, the contrast of particle and field of vibrations is more fundamental in the world of nature than such contrasts as space and time, or past, present, and future, which are the sort of contrasts that our language imposes upon us. The Hopi aspect-contrast... being obligatory upon their verb forms, practically forces the Hopi to notice and observe vibratory phenomena, and furthermore encourages them to find names for and to classify such phenomena. (Whorf 1956, pp.55–56)

In his paper 'A linguistic consideration of thinking in primitive communities', Whorf provides a very convincing argument that so-called 'primitive' communities are, in fact, far from being inferior to 'civilized' societies in their mental functioning, but rather show a higher and more complex level of rational thinking. At the end of the article the author concludes that 'English compared to Hopi is like a bludgeon to a rapier' (Whorf 1956, p.85).

Language as filter

Whorf considers that language, for all its importance in structuring the reality, is in some sense 'a superficial embroidery upon deeper processes of consciousness, which are necessary before any communication, signaling, or symbolism whatsoever can occur' (1956, p.239). The way we 'break up the flux of experience' (Whorf 1956) into static objects is different in different languages. As soon as we 'project the linguistic patterns on the universe' we *see* them there, whether they correspond to reality or not. So first we sort out perceptions (shaping them into concepts) and then label them accordingly. The conceptual representations that develop through learning are related arbitrarily to the perceptual states that activate them (Barsalou 1999).

New concepts are needed. For example in particle physics, our present language is not equipped to describe certain phenomena, the reason being we do not understand them yet and have not developed new concepts. So we have to use inadequate labels to depict something we have not grasped fully yet, thus making the description incomplete.

How can we describe a particle, say, electron, that is both a particle and a wave, or it is neither a particle nor a wave? Either description is inadequate, but we have not worked out a concept yet to grasp the two complementary facets of the electron: under certain circumstances it behaves like a particle, but there are circumstances where it is appropriate to use the wave concept. We need a concept that encompasses both (and we have not developed it yet). Or let us take another example – 'electron spin' that is a different 'spin' from what is conventionally understood because the electron has to spin around *twice* to get back to where it started. So, we need a concept to reflect this peculiarity, and conventional 'spin'-label is inadequate.

The further we go, the more problems arise. For instance, if we want to measure an electron's properties, such as the position and momentum, we find it is impossible in principle to get precise results for *both*. If we measure the position, we cannot be sure of its momentum, and vice versa – if we measure its momentum, we cannot be certain where the electron is. The more we know about the wave aspect of reality, the less we know about the particle, and vice versa. This is known as uncertainty principle. If it was not enough, there are problems with devising experiments. Elementary particles behave differently under observation. The physicists are aware that it is meaningless to ask what the atoms are doing when we are not looking at them, and all we can do is to calculate the probability that each particular experiment will produce a particular result.

All these concepts of uncertainty, complementarity, probability and the disturbance of the system being observed (known collectively as the 'Copenhagen interpretation') are rooted in our traditional scientific approach which does not work in the quantum world. We still have no idea of what elementary particles are really like and what they are doing when we are not looking at them.

Sensory perception → **Different concepts** → **Necessity to label them**

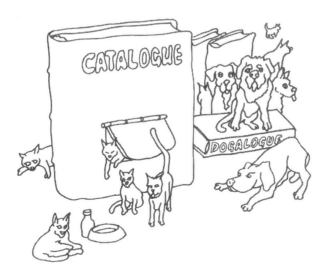

It is a two-way process, and language influences perceptions, too. Anything that does not exist in language goes unnoticed by the majority. Language helps to manage emotional states as well. A 'language filter' protects verbal thinkers from emotional overload. If this filter is absent, the impact of emotional involvement is much greater (Daria 2008).

What is more, language eventually does influence the behaviour of those who speak it, sometimes negatively.

Language may be a very powerful weapon. You can hurt a person with a single word, or destroy someone's life. The author of the Alex Rider series, Anthony Horowitz, remarks that these days a single misplaced sentence can destroy a career and even a life – if someone, anyone, would see anything offensive in it (Horowitz 2007). It is not even necessary to say anything – simply being accused of being disrespectful/offensive can destroy your reputation. You don't have to go very far to find hundreds (thousands?) of examples – Internet blogs, fora, discussion groups just one click away. For example, in one of the discussions, the participants bent backwards to accommodate one very loud 'autism advocate'; they asked the person what they should do in this or that situation not to offend anyone, but they asked only for one condition – to agree to disagree. The result? In minutes, the internet was flooded with complaints from the 'offended': 'This shameful, disrespectful, offensive so-and-so said that they did not care what autistics say! He insulted me!!!' As a consequence, from that day on, hundreds of people who had not known the 'shameful, disrespectful person' dismissed him as their 'enemy'.

It is a very dangerous tendency to impose our own meaning onto words, changing perceptions and making people see what is not there.[7] Unfortunately, PC do-gooders would see offence in everything and anything, and insist on banning dozens of words because of their 'offensive character'. Funnily enough, before the ban, very few people could see *anything offensive* in 'Baa, baa, black sheep', or 'Three Little Pigs', 'blacklisting', or 'brainstorming'.

We should not forget that language is arbitrary; it means we agree what words mean. If we believe the sky should be called red, the sky will be red for us; belief alters experience. When we impose different (and often negative) meaning to 'neutral' words, in effect, we influence perception and alter experience. We also make people think and behave differently. Tell someone 100 times that he is a pig, and he will go 'oink-oink'. (I apologize to the pig, and to anyone who would think that this might be applied to them!)

Children acquire 'cultural-linguistic categories' as they share the experiences of the people around them and thus enter the culture into which they are born. Feral children reared by animals acquire their adoptive parents' ways of communicating and viewing the world.

Although there are language universals common to all verbal languages, these universals are reflected in each language differently. We use language to categorize, analyse and communicate our experiences and our understanding of the world, thus effectively rearranging the 'raw data' into established concepts, labelling them accordingly. Therefore we may speak about the linguistic world of each culture.

So far, the validity of the Sapir-Whorf hypothesis has neither been sufficiently proved nor refuted. Most supporters of this hypothesis are those who studied languages very different in their morphology, syntax, lexicology and structure in general from the Indo-European languages (e.g. Hoijer 1953; Kluckhohn 1954; Thompson 1950). Kluckhohn and Leighton (1946) describe tremendous translation difficulties between English and the Navaho language, concluding that the two languages, in fact, almost literally operate in different worlds. For example Navaho verbs indicate only that people participate or get involved in activities, rather than initiating them; it is reflected in the fatefulness of

Navaho mythology and their passivity and general restlessness (Hoijer 1953).

At present, the work of Whorf has received a renewed interest. Some researchers have developed experiments and methods to test empirically some of the key notions and issues raised by Whorf with intriguing and convincing results that do indicate that different languages shape the way we think.[8]

One of the most prominent critics of Whorf's ideas is the psycholinguist Steven Pinker. In his book *The Language Instinct* (1994/2000) Pinker attempts to debunk Whorf's interpretation of the Hopi notions of time and space and the principle of relativity. One of Pinker's arguments is that Whorf is 'an inspector for the Hartford Fire Insurance Company and an amateur scholar of Native American languages', and not a linguist. It is true that Whorf did not have a PhD in linguistics, but his achievements in the field and the ideas he generated far surpassed those produced by many 'real linguists' in my own and many others' view.[9] If this matter of qualifications were one of the main 'scientific' flaws of Whorf's ideas, it would be laughable. But there are more 'scientific' criticisms of (and unscientific attacks on) Whorf's work, for example, when Pinker writes scathingly: 'no one is really sure how Whorf came up with his outlandish claims, but his limited, badly analyzed sample of Hopi speech and his long-term leanings towards mysticism must have helped' (Pinker 1994/2000, p.63).

To illustrate a 'good' analysis of Hopi speech, Pinker cites the work of Ekkehart Malotki (1983) to show that Hopis do indeed have time terms. After a thorough analysis, Professor Dan Moonhawk Alford (2002), however, questions Malotki's conclusions and illustrates obvious drawbacks of Malotki's research (Alford 1994, 2002).[10]

Another critic of the Sapir-Whorf hypothesis, Stevan Harnad has put forward his own psychophysical hypothesis to prove that all languages are intertranslatable. In fact, he defines language as 'an approximately intertranslatable system for approximately categorizing the world' (Harnad 1996, p.34). Intertranslatability, Harnad admits, is never exact, it is always approximate; and categorization, like translation, is also approximate rather than exact (Harnad 1987). However, approximation can be made as close as one desires, perhaps using a profligate quantity of words but with the resultant meaning coming as close as need be, reducing uncertainty in the shared external communicative context (Steklis and Harnad 1976). Harnad's theory is primarily a bottom-up psychophysical model for representation of word meaning. Psychophysics[11] poses the following questions: (1) What stimuli can we detect? (2) What stimuli can we tell apart (discriminate)? (3) What stimuli can we identify (categorize)? Harnad does not see any problems with the first two questions because they concern the sensitivity of our sense receptors, though he does admit that the limits of our ability to make sensory discriminations will also influence our ability to make conceptual and semantic distinctions.

One of the earliest critics of the Whorf hypothesis, a social philosopher Feuer (1953) duly stated that one would not expect people speaking different languages to have different ways of perceiving space, time, causation and other fundamental elements of the physical world because a correct perception of these elements is necessary to survival. Correct perception was not defined; it was assumed that all humans possess it.

However, if we deal with sensory perceptual abilities in autism, we definitely encounter problems with these 'easy' questions. Some autistic individuals can (and do) detect stimuli to which 'normal' individuals are blind, deaf and so forth. Here are just a few examples:

> Some of the energy-saver fluorescent light bulbs have such a high degree of flicker that...some people on the spectrum feel like they are standing in the middle of a disco nightclub. (Grandin 2008, p.60)

> I have an acute sense of color. I see rainbows in a piece of ice, some colors and lights have sent me into manic and euphoric episodes and giggle fits. (Williams 2007)

> [The] sound sensitivity [on some frequencies] was so odd that
> I did not recognise it because I felt it as vibrations rather than
> as noise. (Blackman 2001, p.200)

Or there may be the opposite, when they experience hyposensitivity
and do not see, hear or feel certain stimuli, for instance:

> My senses would sometimes become dull to the point that I
> could not clearly see or hear, and the world around me would
> seemingly cease to exist. (Hawthorne 2002)

There are other sensory perceptual problems as well, such as
fragmented perception:

> I had a fragmented perception of things at the best of times,
> seeing eyes or a nose or whiskers or a mouth but mostly
> putting the bits together in my head. (Williams 1999a,
> p.162)

Distortions can also be an issue:

> To some...individuals [with visual processing problems] the
> world looks like it is viewed through a kaleidoscope: flat,
> without depth perception, and broken into pieces. For others,
> it is like looking through a small tube, seeing only the small
> circle of vision directly in front of them, with no peripheral
> vision. (Grandin 2008, p.78)

> I sometimes was seeing my hands and the things I was
> touching as if they were multiples...[the] image was either
> multiplied, or overlaid by similar reproductions of itself in
> duplicate. (Blackman 2001, p.268)

Another argument supposed to 'kill' the Whorf hypothesis is
the universality of colour perception.[12] Brown and Lennenberg
(1954) reported their experiment that showed that differences in
ability to recognize and remember colours were associated with
the availability of 'colour-names'. Berlin and Kay (1969) studied

colour terms in several languages. They found that although languages did differ in how they subdivided the light spectrum, the effects on colour perception seemed minimal. However, it is possible to hypothesize that the 'nameless colours' can be ignored as 'unimportant'. It has been found that although the boundaries of colour categories are established by the physiology of the colour receptors, these boundaries show some plasticity and can be moved depending on subcategorization and naming alone (Bornstein 1987). Here we deal with 'acquired distinctiveness' and 'acquired similarity' of cues: two stimuli would look more alike if they have the same name and more different if they had different names (Gibson 1969; Lawrence 1950). As Miller puts it, 'many of the differences we perceive among things and events would not be noticed if society had not forced us to learn that they have different names' (Miller 1951, p.199). Yet again, the situation may be even more complicated in autism. Some autistic individuals do see colours differently, for example:

> I still have troubles, especially with colors. It is not that I don't see colors, it is that I see wrong colors. The worst ones are colors made of two other colors because instead of seeing one color I see a mix of the two other colors and I have to figure out exactly what color I am looking at. An example of this…is if I look at purple I see swirling reds and blues. This doesn't bother my eyes (in fact sometimes it looks pretty kewl) but it does bother my brain when I am trying to see the one single color. (McKean 1999)

Bearing all these differences in perception in mind, we can hardly talk about similar detection and discrimination of stimuli (the first two 'easy' questions of Harnad's first mentioned on p.102). Harnad's third question, about identification and categorization, is about the naming of sensory categories – which is at the heart of the Sapir-Whorf hypothesis: our language influences the way we see reality. Harnad argues that it is the other way round – reality influences language, so that 'we tend to have names for the kinds of things that we think there are and that we tend to talk about; if the existence of new things is pointed out, we can always baptize them with a new name' (Harnad 1996, p.32).

People use language to classify the world in a shared and modifiable way. Swapping the meaning of words is also swapping experiences (Harnad 1996). The problem starts when we do *not* share experiences, which is very common in autism. For example, how many people will share Lucy Blackman's experiences described here?

> When I had thought about my body or the world immediately around me, I had visualised it much as I saw it, as composites of smaller composites, with a fairly arbitrary relationship between the various odds and ends. (Blackman 2001, p.265)

> I...was beginning to understand that I was using my language to make a link with people who lived on another planet in terms of what their senses told them. (Blackman 2001, p.186)

Back to Harnad's third question. Harnad suggests that learning to categorize requires three kinds of internal representation: (1) 'iconic representations' (i.e. physical patterns that concrete objects project onto the surfaces of our sensory receptors); (2) 'categorical representations' which preserve and encode only invariant sensory properties *shared* by all the members of a concrete perceptual category; and (3) 'symbolic representations' which are the names for the categories that have iconic and categorical representations (Harnad 1996; emphasis is mine).

Acquiring all these three representations may be a slow process in autism as individuals with autism have to go through several stages to 'get to the final picture' (i.e. the functionality of an object), for instance:

> When I am confronted with a hammer, I am initially confronted...with a number of unrelated parts: I notice a

cubical piece of iron...[and] a coincidental bar-like piece of wood. After that, I am struck by the coincidental nature of the iron and the wooden thing resulting in the unifying perception of a hammer-like configuration. The name 'hammer' is not immediately within reach but appears when configuration has been sufficiently stabilized over time. Finally, the use of a tool becomes clear. (VanDalen 1995, p.11)

Similar experiences have been described by other individuals with autism, as well. Moving through several stages to reach comprehension of objects and their functions can be complicated by associative thinking, which seems to be quite typical for autistic people (Grandin 1996a; Williams 1996). For example, when Tito enters a room for the first time, before he recognizes that a door is a door, he sees the colour; if he defines the colour as 'yellow', in his mind he immediately lines up all the yellow things he knows; then he moves on to a rectangular shape of the door, then to levers and hinges, and only having analysed all these features (a yellow rectangular shape with levers and hinges that allows one to come inside the room) Tito safely reaches a conclusion and completes his labelling – it's a door (Mukhopadhyay 2008).

Non-verbal languages

We have to make another very important point here. Though non-verbal autistic individuals lack verbal language, it does not mean they have no language at all. Let us look at the definition of *language* (p.90) again. It is conventional to identify symbols in this definition as words. The error of mistaking the acoustic or written manifestation of language (reflected in speech) for language itself leads to the misconception that language is necessarily verbal. However, though it is unconventional to propose it, verbal (linguistic) words are not the only signs or symbols that satisfy the criteria of language. It is logical, therefore, to distinguish two types of languages – verbal (consisting of words) and non-verbal (consisting of non-verbal symbols). Autistic children, like non-autistic ones, learn through interaction with the world, but their reality is very different. They learn their language(s) through interaction with objects and people on the sensory level. That is why their 'words' have nothing to do with the conventional names for things and events that we use to describe the function of these things and events. Their 'words' are literal, they store sensations produced by objects through interaction, and they 'name' them accordingly.

> Going back to the door before it is known in terms of function; before it is, in fact, 'door' (which is a function concept), it may have no word at all. Later, as one moves from non-physical sensing of what happens to be a door to a physical-based sensing of what happens to be a door, its sound-concept is very unlikely to be 'door'. If you tapped the door, it may (depending on the door) tell you its name is 'took'. If it made a noise when it gave way under impact, it might say its name is 'rerr' if it drags on the carpet or 'ii-er' depending on the sound of the hinges. It may have no sound concept at all or sound concept relating to the experience of door might come from the emotional experience of sensory buzz associated with that door. So taking the example of the swinging door fascination, if the buzz experience brought out a little suppressed squeal (hard to write [it] in letters)... the sound concept associated with the experience of door may well become this stored and later triggered sound. [Or if] the buzz experience brought out an emotionally connected body expression movement such as sudden staccato contraction of the fingers into outward-facing fists that jerk suddenly back towards the torso, this may become stored as something akin to a language sign associated with the buzz experience brought on by the swinging door. (Williams 1998, pp.99–100)

One sense (sometimes several senses) becomes dominant for storing memories, developing 'language(s)' and constructing thoughts, for example, 'My dominant sensory channel is hearing. It dominates to such an extent that I dream in sounds most of the time, even when I sleep at night. So if anyone asks me, "What did you see in your dream?" I would answer, "I hear my dream"" (Mukhopadhyay 2008, p.196).

Even if some autistic individuals cannot communicate through conventional systems, such as talking, typing and so on, they still have a form of inner language. Here we may distinguish several 'sensory-based languages':

1. *Visual language:* Individuals use visual images.

2. *Tactile language:* Individuals recognize things by touching them, feeling textures and surfaces with their hands, bare feet, or their cheeks. Through touch they acquire information about the size and shape of things, but not about their function or purpose. They store the information for later reference and may find similar objects (e.g. a plastic ball and a rubber ball) to be completely different 'words' in their vocabulary because they *feel* different.

3. *Kinaesthetic language:* Individuals learn about things and events through the physical movements of their body. Each thing or activity is identified by certain pattern of body movement. They know places and distances by the amount and pattern of the movement.

4. *Auditory language:* Individuals remember objects and events by 'sound pictures'. If the object is 'silent', they may tap it to recognize it by the sound it produces.

5. *Smell language:* Objects and people are identified by smell.

6. *Taste language:* Individuals may lick objects and people to feel the taste they give on the tongue.[13]

No wonder that spoken words are often perceived as mere sounds. It is difficult to sense or feel a ball, for example, in the auditory frame 'ball'. Autistic individuals may not recognize the thing if given its verbal (conventional) name, but may easily identify it with the sound it produces while bouncing, the smell or the feel on the hand. Each individual may use one or several 'languages' to make sense about the world. Given perceptual differences, including sensory perceptual problems (fragmentation, hyper- or hyposensitivities, etc.) one or several systems may become inconsistent and/or meaningless, and they have to use those that are reliable (different for different individuals) to check the information they are flooded with. Each individual has a unique sensory perceptual profile and has acquired (voluntarily or involuntarily) compensations and strategies to recognize things and make sense of the world. One and the same person may use different systems at different times, depending on many factors that can influence the 'perceptual quality', such as stress, fatigue, 'environmental sensory pollution' (bright lights, noise) and the like.

The difficulty interpreting these languages is rooted in our own verbal language. In order to examine very different languages we tend to think in terms of our own tongue (Whorf 1956). Just as our 'normal' perception interferes with our understanding of other possible sensory experiences, our verbal language imposes 'normal' established categories, thus hindering our comprehension of other possible interpretations.

At the end of his paper 'The Origin of Words: A Psychophysical Hypothesis' (1996), Harnad poses a question: could two symbolic representational systems fail to be intertranslatable? He answers with a firm 'No'. However, in the case of 'autistic languages' compared with 'normal verbal languages', 'intertranslatability' is unlikely, because of lack of a *shared experience* which is essential for any translatability. For example:

> I don't think that what I see is what you see. That is unless what you see are vague clouds and shadows of substance. (McKean 1999)

> [Some autistics] may see colors with no clear shapes. Sometimes they report that images break up into pieces like a mosaic. (Grandin 2008, p.186)

Unbelievably I lived in a world (and still do) where the environment of our Earth, with its consistent gravity, sound waves and refracted light, was but an invention of fiction writers. (Blackman 2001, p.155)

What I do realise is that I do not see the world as others do. Most people take the routines of life and everyday connections for granted. The fact they can see, hear, smell, touch and relate to others is 'normal'. For me, these things are often painfully overwhelming, non-existent or just confusing. (Lawson 1998, pp.2–3)

As we have seen, although the Sapir-Whorf hypothesis (that our ways of perceiving and interpreting the world are formed by the categories of the language we speak) is not considered proved and has been criticized, it seems to be applicable to verbal compared with (autistic) 'non-verbal languages' – they do conceptualize the world in different ways. Whorf's suggestion that we cut nature up, organize it into concepts and give significances the way we do, mostly because we are all in an agreement that is coded in the patterns of our language, not because nature itself is segmented in exactly that way for all to see – is very telling in the case at hand. All conceptual systems are relative (Whorf 1956).[14]

If different intelligent systems have different perceptual systems, the developed conceptual systems may also differ. Because their symbols contain different perceptual content, they may refer to different structures in the world and may not be functionally equivalent (Barsalou 1999). Non-verbal and verbal languages dissect nature in different ways. The 'sensory concepts' acquired by an autistic child 'speaking' one (or several) non-verbal languages do not represent 'shared knowledge'. However, the child uses these categories and the relations between them to understand the world.

Cultural exchange involves the sharing or swapping of different forms of the language and ways of interpretation all of which have arisen from essentially the same sensory, perceptual and cognitive mechanisms. Yet, hard as one might try, it may be much easier for a human being with interpretation [i.e. non-autistic] to have a cultural exchange with an octopus with interpretation than it may be for a person with interpretation to comprehend someone who functions without it, primarily on the level of sensing [i.e. autistic]. (Williams 1998, p.107)

So, there *are* languages that are *not* 'intertranslatable' – in the terminology of Donna Williams: the language of sensing and the language of interpretation. She outlines this in more detail as follows:

> Both on the level of verbal language, facial expression, body language and signing, the language of the system of sensing does not conform to the rules of the language of interpretation and it would be irrational to expect it to. (Williams 1998, p.102)

> I struggled to use 'the world' language to describe a way of thinking and being and experiencing for which this world gives you no words or concepts. (Williams 1999c, p.77)

Yet, those who share the sensory-based language understand each other perfectly well, irrespective of what cultures they were born in:

> Language and concepts within the system of sensing are repeated again and again by people devoid of interpretation or in whom interpretation is an inconsistent and secondary system who live on other sides of the earth and have never met each other. (Williams 1998, p.102)

Restrictions of linguistic systems

Whorf urges us to study many languages to improve our thinking and own use of language. It will give us many different perspectives of reality. However, the more we rely on verbal language, the more we go away from reality as it is. Don Juan in Castaneda (1974) compares 'normal' perception with a 'bubble' formed around us so we perceive only the reflection of our own world view. To open the 'bubble' would be to suspend the description and experience reality without conceptual baggage. It will help us get a glimpse of the world free from imposed meanings, culture and language.

'Normal' perceptions of the outside world are clouded by the verbal notions and concepts in terms of which people do their thinking. All things are converted into signs for the more intelligible abstractions of human invention. But in doing this, 'normal' people rob the objects and experiences they label of a great deal of their native thinghood (Huxley 1956/2004).

Though himself a supreme master of language, Goethe understood too well the restrictions any linguistic system imposes on people:

> We talk too much... I personally should like to renounce speech altogether and, like organic Nature, communicate everything I have to say in sketches. That fig tree, this little snake, the cocoon on my window sill quietly awaiting its future – all these are momentous signatures... There is something futile, mediocre, even...floppish about speech. By contrast, how the gravity of Nature and her silence startle you, when you stand face to face with her, undistracted... (Goethe, cited in Huxley 1954/2004, p.22)

Ralph Abraham explores the role of language in human functioning and come to the conclusion that:

> When [verbal] language began we lost our connection with the natural world. (p.36) Verbal language is poorly adapted to space/time patterns. (p.37) We try to map experience into language, but we must admit that in mapping it into language, into a popular process, we strip it of 90 percent of its meaning (p.136). (Abraham in Sheldrake *et al.* 2005)

> People tell us from the time we are born that the world is such and such and so and so, and naturally we have no choice

but to accept that the world is the way people have been telling us. (Castaneda 1998, p.103)

In this context, the Sapir-Whorf hypothesis appears to be valid. The reality we believe really exists depends on how we name things and describe them in language. Language seems to create a linguistically restricted mind with (rigid) conceptual intelligence, in contrast to the fluid intelligence of an unrestricted mind.

Huxley urged us as humans to intensify our ability to look at the world directly and not through the medium of concepts, which 'distorts every given fact into the all too familiar likeliness of some generic label or explanatory abstraction' (Huxley 1954/2004, p.22). In his fascinating essay, Huxley cites the line of William Blake which inspired the title of his work: 'If the doors of perception were cleansed everything would appear to man as it is, infinite.' Huxley compares his experiences of 'cleansed perception' (under the influence of mescalin) with the 'normal perception' that he calls 'our pathetic imbecility' (Huxley 1954/2004, p.19).

Being verbal thinkers, non-autistic individuals tend never to pay much attention to their sensory environment. Temple Grandin says that non-autistic humans 'are abstractified in their sensory perception as well as their thoughts... Animals and autistic humans don't see their ideas of things; they see the actual things themselves' (Grandin and Johnson 2005, p.30). With age, non-autistic people's perception becomes even less accurate. Every time they look at something they just pick up a few features and they recognize the whole picture from their past experiences and memories. Unlike autistic individuals, non-autistics see more from the 'inside', from what is in their heads (from what they *think* is out there), than what is actually there outside of their mental world (Bogdashina 2003, 2004, 2005; Daria 2008). Temple Grandin states that autistic people see the details that make up the world, while non-autistic individuals blur all the details together into their general concept of the world (that is not necessarily a correct one).

To be shaken out of the ruts of ordinary perception, to be shown for a few timeless hours the outer and the inner world, not as they appear to an animal obsessed with survival or to a human being obsessed with words and notions, but as they are apprehended, directly and unconditionally, by Mind at Large – thus an experience of inestimable value to everyone and especially to the intellectual. (Huxley 1954/2004, p.46)

Unrestricted by 'pathetic imbecility'

Can autism help 'normal' people to have a glimpse of this 'cleansed perception', unrestricted by the 'pathetic imbecility'? We are able to reconstruct what cleansed perception is and get some idea of alternative consciousness by analysis of the research studies and personal accounts of individuals with autism, combined with experiences of 'normal' individuals under atypical circumstances.[15]

Dunbar (1996) argues that human language evolved initially as a specific social tool for negotiating interpersonal relationships, for naming and talking about other people and their concerns. Mithen (1996, cited in Humphrey 1998) agrees, suggesting that the 'linguistic module' of the brain was originally available to the module of 'social intelligence', not to the modules of 'technical' and 'natural history' intelligence.

Stern (1985) suggests that infants' initial interpersonal knowledge is mainly unsharable, amodal and instance-specific. Language changes all that by fracturing the amodal global experience of the child and estranging the infant from direct contact with their personal experience. Language creates a space between interpersonal experience: as lived and as represented. On the other hand language provides a tool to a child to share their personal experience of the world with others (Stern 1985).

Lack (or delayed acquisition) of language (typical in autism) seems to allow better awareness and an extraordinary memory capability. The connection between lack of verbal language and a good memory is illustrated by the research study of memory of humans and chimps. Professor Tetsuro Matsuzawa and colleagues pitted five-year-old chimps and human undergraduates in a series of memory tests. Both groups were briefly shown numbers from 1 to 9 on a touch-screen monitor; they had to remember where on the screen each number appeared, and the chimpanzees beat the humans (Inoue and Matsuzawa 2007; Matsuzawa 2009).

It is interesting to note that there is a big similarity between savant skills (especially in art and music) and the talents emerging in older people who develop temporal-frontal lobe dementia. Dr Bruce Miller at the University of California in San Francisco, who has studied these patients for many years, describes cases of individuals who acquire artistic and musical skills as their language deteriorates (Miller *et al.* 1998, 2000).

Lorna Selfe (1977) who worked with Nadia, an autistic savant, hypothesizes that it was Nadia's language – or rather her failure to develop it – that was the key to explain her extraordinary ability to draw. Selfe believes that it was Nadia's lack of conceptualization that allowed her to see everything around her the way it really was, not as categorized things. The girl could match different items with the same perceptual quality, but she failed to match items belonging to the same conceptual class (Selfe 1985). For Nadia, everything was 'the' something, not 'a' horse, for example, but 'the' horse she had seen, remembered and reproduced on paper. Selfe (1983) examined several other autistic individuals with outstanding graphic skills and came to the same conclusion:

> It is therefore proposed that without the hypothesized domination of language and verbal mediation in the early years when graphic competence was acquired, these subjects were able to attend to the spatial characteristics of their optic array and to represent these aspects in their drawing... These children therefore have a more direct access to visual imagery in the sense that their drawings are not so strongly 'contaminated' by the usual 'designating and naming' properties of normal children's drawings. (p.201)

For non-autistic individuals it is the object labels (concepts) that are of ultimate importance, as they give us the idea of what is there without any need to be aware of all the details (a few are enough to identify an object). We are blinded by our 'mental paradigms' or 'mindsets' (Snyder 1996). This can be illustrated by 'normal' children's drawings. They draw what they can verbally identify, that is, they draw not what they see but what they know is there, their own 'internalised schema for objects' (Snyder and Thomas 1997). For example, they draw a person or an animal primitively, devoid of details. In contrast, autistic artists (having no mental 'restraints') draw their pictures with minute details, without filtering significant from insignificant information. They do not impose either linguistic concepts or expectations on their work and consequently, to them, every detail is of equal importance (Snyder 1996). Their perception is more accurate because the interpretation does not interfere with or distort what is perceived:

> No normal preschool child has been known to draw naturalistically. Autism is apparently a necessary condition for a preschool child to draw an accurate detail of natural scenes. (Snyder and Thomas 1997, p.95)

When at the age of eight Nadia (after intensive teaching) acquired some language, her drawing abilities partly diminished.[16] Elizabeth Newson summarizes the outcome in her Postscript to Selfe's book about Nadia:

> Nadia seldom draws spontaneously now, although from time to time one of her horses appears on a steamed up window. If asked, however, she will draw: particularly portraits... In style [these] are much more economical than her earlier drawings, with much less detail... The fact that Nadia at eight and nine can produce recognizable drawings of the people around her still makes her talent a remarkable one for her age; but one would no longer say that it is unbelievable...
>
> If the partial loss of her gift is the price that must be paid for language – even just enough language to bring her

into some kind of community of discourse with her small protected world – we must, I think, be prepared to pay that price on Nadia's behalf. (Newson 1977, p.129)

Having compared the similarity between savant skills in art and music and the talents emerging in patients with temporal-frontal lobe dementia, Temple Grandin has developed a theory that both skills may be explained by the person having direct access to the visual or musical parts of the brain. Grandin suggests that potentially *all* humans have these skills but the use of language masks their ability to access them:

> In my own case, I can think in pictures without words. I can access my visual memory directly because it is not masked by verbal words. When I read, I instantly translate what I read into pictures. From my own experience, I can agree with the idea that people with autism directly access primary parts of the brain that are not accessible to verbal thinkers. (Grandin 2008, p.190)

Grandin's idea is supported by Margaret Bauman's research with brain autopsies that shows that the parts of the brain where procedural memories (not requiring words) are stored are intact in people with autism (Bauman and Kemper 1994, 2005).

Thinking without language

Some scholars still insist that (verbal) language is essential for intelligence (e.g. Dennett 1994). According to this limited view, lack of (verbal) language means inability to think. Such researchers argue that animals act on instinct only.[17] Dennett criticizes the views of Merlin Donald (1991) who argues that 'thinking without language' is not necessarily primitive and can be remarkably sophisticated. To support his claim, Donald gives several examples, one of them being the capabilities of congenitally deaf individuals who (for whatever reasons) have not yet required any language. Dennett insists, however, that language-less thought in humans is impossible – all humans, including the deaf who have not developed any sign language, are still beneficiaries of the shaping role of language, and might have structures in their brains that are direct products of the language that most of their ancestors in recent millennia have shared (Dennett 1994). It would have been just a theoretical discussion if there had not been very important implications. If verbal language is essential for human thinking, how can we categorize those autistic individuals whose cognitive functioning is perceptually based? Shall we deny them the ability to think? How shall we categorize the work by, for example, Temple Grandin, who is a visual thinker?

> My experience as a visual thinker with autism makes it clear to me that thought does not have to be verbal...to be real. I considered my thoughts to be real long before I learned that there was a difference between visual and verbal thinkers. I am not saying that animals and normal humans and autistics think alike. But I do believe that recognising different capacities and kinds of thought and expression can lead to greater connectedness and understanding. (Grandin 1996a, p.164)

Research (Farah 1989; Zeki 1992) shows that verbal thought and visual thinking work via different brain systems. In general, research has shown that there is abnormal processing of verbal language in autism. For instance, Just *et al.* (2004) have investigated sentence comprehension in autism and found that compared with controls, high-functioning autistic individuals exhibited lower levels of activation in Broca's area and higher levels of activation in Wernicke's area.[18] Just *et al.* (2004) have suggested that there may be underconnectivity among cortical areas. In addition, neuroimaging research (Koshino *et al.* 2005) shows a tendency in autism to use visual-spatial regions of the brain to compensate for higher-order cortical regions. To support these research findings many papers refer to or quote Temple Grandin, whose insightful book *Thinking in Pictures* (1996a) and numerous articles describe visual thinking in detail, for example:

> I think in pictures. Words are like a second language to me. I translate both spoken and written words into full-color movies, complete with sound, which run like a VCR tape in my head... Language-based thinkers often find this phenomenon difficult to understand. (Grandin 1996b, p.3)

Another recent study (Kana *et al.* 2006) has examined the performance of high-functional individuals with autism in a task that required the integration of the visuospatial, language and cognitive processing. They used two types of sentences: low-imagery sentences (e.g. 'Addition, subtraction and multiplication are all math skills') and high imagery sentences (e.g. 'The number eight when rotated 90 degrees looks like a pair of eyeglasses'). The control group activated parietal and occipital brain regions associated with imagery primarily in the high-imagery condition while using more inferior frontal language regions when processing low-imagery sentences. In contrast, the autism group showed imagery-related activation for comprehending both the low- and high-imagery sentences, suggesting that they were using mental imagery in both conditions. The results indicate that autistic individuals were using what Temple Grandin calls 'thinking in pictures' much of the time (Kana *et al.* 2006). It has been suggested that autistic individuals may think in visuospatial ways to compensate for their language deficits (Hermelin and O'Connor 1990; O'Connor and Hermelin 1987).

Visualized thinking patterns vary from person to person. Some 'visualizers' (like Temple Grandin, for example) can easily search memory pictures as if they were searching through slides and are able to control the rate at which images appear in their mind. Others have great difficulty in controlling the rate and may end up overloaded, with too many images coming all at once. Still others are slow to interpret the information in their 'visual mode' and may have problems with visualizing quickly what is said, or mentally holding visual images together. Besides, the 'quality' of visual thinking may depend on the state the person is in (Bogdashina 2004).

Though the visuospatial system has traditionally been considered as an intact area (or even enhanced ability) in autism (based on the relatively high scores on the Block Design and the embedded figures tests) (Goldstein *et al.* 2001; Happe 1999; Jolliffe and Baron-Cohen 1997; Shah and Frith 1993; Siegel, Minshew and Goldstein 1996), there is evidence that not all autistic individuals use their visuospatial regions for cognitive functioning. Those with visual processing problems (fragmentation, distortions, etc.) compensate by using other sensory modalities instead. For example: 'Unlike Temple, I do NOT think in pictures. I imagine primarily in feel, movement, kinaesthetic and via acoustics made by the object when struck. I "visualise" like a blind person' (Williams 2003b, p.2).

Notes

1. Sometimes it is referred to as the Whorf hypothesis of the principle of linguistic relativity, but it is only fair to acknowledge the influence of Sapir on the development of the theory.

2. Benjamin Lee Whorf (1897–1941) was an outstanding scholar in linguistics. A very interesting fact is that he did not train for it. He was educated as a chemical engineer and turned out to become a very good one. His engineering skills provided him with a framework for researching languages which became his obsessive interest. In addition to his remarkable career as a chemical engineer whose expertise was eagerly sought by chemical manufacturers, and his scholarly linguistic work that was equal to that of many full-time researchers, Whorf was a brilliant businessman who was able to attract business to the company he worked for. It is truly remarkable that one person could achieve distinction in several separate kinds of work (Carroll 1956). Not everyone knows that Whorf's interest in linguistics was rooted in religion. As if his work in engineering, his linguistic research and his many community activities were not enough, Whorf found time to pursue his other interests, including psychology, anthropology, botany, astrology and diary writing.

    Whorf's meeting with Edward Sapir (1884–1939), a highly recognized authority in the field of linguistics, had a great impact on the development of Whorf's linguistic talent.

With a fashion at present to give a retrospective diagnosis of autism to outstanding personalities of the past, Whorf would be a very good candidate for this.

Lack of interest in social activities: Whorf was happy to stay alone if he could spend all his time researching and working on the project he was interested in. He liked the company of those with similar interests and always had something novel and interesting to say on the subject of the discussion. One of his students recalled: 'Whorf was a quiet, contemplative teacher; he would not stop at remaining silent for a seemingly interminable time searching his mind to recall something or to think through a problem' (Chase 1956, p.22).

The ability to concentrate and obsessive interests: Whatever Whorf did, he was capable of very deep concentration on a subject; the rest of the world just faded away.

Perfectionism and meticulousness: All his manuscripts were nearly error-free, in neat handwriting.

Lack of ambitions and vanity: Though he enrolled for a doctorate programme of studies at the Yale University, he did it to pursue his intellectual interests, not to obtain formal degrees. Whorf was very generous in sharing his remarkable perspectives and ideas with others (Chase 1956).

3. Whorf describes the Hopi culture and life style:

> A peaceful agricultural society isolated by geographic features and nomad enemies in a land of scanty rainfall, arid agriculture that could be made successful only by the utmost perseverance (hence the value of persistence and repetition), necessity for collaboration (hence emphasis on the psychology of teamwork and on mental factors in general), corn and rain as primary criteria of value, need of extensive PREPARATIONS and precautions to assure crops in the poor soil and precarious climate, keen realization of dependence upon nature favoring prayer and a religious attitude toward the forces of nature, especially prayer and religion directed towards the ever-needed blessing, rain – these things interacted with Hopi linguistic patterns to mold them, to be molded again by them, and so little by little to shape the Hopi world-outlook. (Whorf 1956, p.157)

4. Carlos Castaneda (1925–1998), an anthropologist, wrote 12 books which were presented as real-life accounts of being an apprentice of Don Juan Matus, a Yaqui shaman, and of the other practices and knowledge of Yaqui shamanism. Castaneda's work was critically acclaimed and considered authentical until 1976 when a number of works appeared containing strong criticisms and accusations of deception and plagiarism (see, e.g. DeMille

1976; Fikes 1993; Noel 1976). Castaneda's critics point out internal inconsistencies in the chronologies of his books, the absence of a Yaqui vocabulary and the close parallel between Castaneda's experiences and those reported in other works on shamanism to prove that his work is, in fact, fiction. His proponents, however, insist that it does not assert that neither Castaneda's knowledge of shamanism is in any way defective, nor that his ability to communicate his personal experiences of shamanic practices is deficient. For example, David Silverman states that any phenomenological account is interesting in its own right: 'It does not matter to me in the least whether any or all of the "events" reported by Castaneda ever "took place," just as it does not matter to Levi-Strauss if his "book on myths is itself a kind of myth"' (Silverman 1975, p.169).

5. Recent research on how different languages shape the way people perceive and think about space and time has confirmed Whorf's original ideas and produced very interesting results (e.g. Levinson and Wilkins 2006). For example, Dr Lera Boroditsky and colleagues (Stanford University) have collected and analysed data from China, Chile, Greece, Russia, Indonesia and Aboriginal Australia. Experiments have shown that the Kuuk Thaayore (a small Aboriginal community in northern Australia) are much better in spatial orientation and navigational ability than the English speakers. The researchers account this to the fact that, unlike the English who define space relative to the speaker using such words as 'right', 'left', 'front', 'back' and so on, the Aboriginal groups employ general direction terms (north, south, east, west) (Levinson and Wilkins 2006). They stay oriented where they are, even in unfamiliar places and buildings. The same terms are used in all the situations, even in relation to trivial objects. For instance, they may say 'Move the spoon to the southsoutheast a little bit' or 'What is it there on your northwest leg?'

Representation of time is closely connected to that of space. In the experiments to establish how different linguistic communities show temporal progression of events, results for the Aboriginal groups depended on the direction the participants were facing: when they were facing south, they arranged the cards (depicting different stages of an event) from left to right, but when they faced the opposite direction, the cards went from right to left (Boroditsky 2009).

6. Whorf insists that no language is 'primitive':

> [T]hough [linguistic] systems differ widely, yet in the order, harmony, and beauty of the systems, and in their respective subtleties and penetrating analysis of reality, all men are equal. This fact is independent of the state of evolution as regards material culture, savagery, civilization, moral or ethical development, etc... [T]he crudest savage may unconsciously manipulate with effortless ease a linguistic system so intricate, manifoldly

systemized, and intellectually difficult that it requires the lifetime study of our greatest scholars to describe its working. (1956, pp.263–264)

7. The situation with 'political correctness' and 'banning offensive words' resembles a dangerous prediction made by George Orwell in his novel *Nineteen Eighty-Four* (1949 / 1987) that shows an official language as one of the weapons to control the public by the authoritarian Big Brother government being Newspeak – the official language of the country. This language not only dictated expression and therefore world-view, but also shaped the mental patterns and made all other modes of thought impossible. Words including justice, freedom, democracy and honour were simply removed from the language, and the remaining ones were stripped of 'undesirable' meanings; for example, the word 'free' could not be used in its old meaning of 'politically or intellectually free', but was allowed in statements such as 'The dog is free from lice' (Orwell 1949/1987, pp.343–344, 349).

8. See, for example, Boroditsky 2009; Levinson 2003.

9. The same 'not a real/amateur linguist argument' has been (and will be?) repeated again and again (see, e.g. professional linguist's mockery of amateurs: Pullum 1991 calls Whorf: 'that fine amateur linguist' (p.160), and a 'Connecticut fire prevention inspector and weekend language-fancier' (p.163). We should all be grateful to physicists who did not hold Einstein's job as a patent officer (a technical assistant-level III at the federal office in Bern, later promoted to technical assistant-level II) against his genius in theoretical physics. Whorf was not that lucky. His choice to keep his day job as a chemical engineer and a businessman while pursuing his passion of studying linguistics was turned against him. Whorf was offered several academic or scholarly positions but refused to accept them. This quote attributed to Einstein seems to explain his decision: 'A practical profession is a salvation for a man of my type: an academic career compels a young man to scientific production, and only strong characters can resist the temptation of superficial analysis.'

10. To illustrate the limitations of Malotki's research, Alford provides transcription of a PBS video series on Mind: Language, where Malotki is shown working with a Hopi speaker – a woman perhaps in her late twenties or early thirties:

> Malotki: Okay, let-let-let's interrupt here for a minute. I just heard one expression… What was that, *kui-vun-sut?*
>
> Hopi: Mm-hum. [clear throat] *Kui-vun-sut.*
>
> Malotki: *Kui-vun-sut.* In other words, to go and pray to the sun with corn meal, and that's why kui-vun-sut, that means the TIME when you do this?

Hopi: Yes, uh-huh. [quietly] The sun's...barely sunrise.

Notice that, in this unequal whiteman-expert/native-woman sociological imbalance, 'Yes...' probably means 'That's the way you would say it,' while *barely sunrise* is the *real* answer. But more important, this documentation of fieldwork then allows narrator George Page to call Whorf 'wrong' a few minutes later – all because of Malotki hearing what he wants to hear ('Yes') instead of the real answer: that the phrase described a particular growing lightening of the morning sky, not our Western abstract notion of time with past, present and future! How does this fieldwork make Whorf 'wrong'? Fifty-some years before Malotki tortured this time-confession out of that poor Hopi woman, Whorf wrote that:

> In Hopi however all phase terms, like 'summer, morning,' etc., are not nouns but a kind of adverb... It means 'when it is morning' or 'while morning-phase is occurring'... Nothing is suggested about time except the perpetual 'getting later' of it. And so there is no basis here for a formless item answering to our 'time'.

Malotki's Hopi consultant actually gives an even better description, having to do with a gradual lightening of the sky characteristic of early morning...

The best is yet to come: Malotki follows quickly with:

> They [Hopis] are living with time at every point of their lives, but not necessarily of course in the way we perceive time today. Before the encounter with the whiteman, there had never been a need for naming hour or minutes or seconds. In the Hopi society, time is probably experienced as a more organic or natural phenomenon.

Maybe it's just me again, but do you see any contradiction between this statement and the previous one? There's 'this phenomenon of time that we all experience', and then there's the Hopi experience of time as 'a more organic or natural phenomenon' – which, ostensibly, we as Westerners don't experience as part of this phenomenon of time that we all experience (Alford 2002).

11. Psychophysics is the branch of psychology that is concerned with our perceptual capacity.

12. One should also mention the 'Eskimo words for snow' argument with the desire to blame Whorf for this 'hoax' (Martin 1986; Pinker 1994/2004; Pullum 1991). While it is fair to blame the media and scholars who do not bother to check the facts for exaggerating the number of words for 'snow' in Eskimo languages (from four to 400) and overgeneralizing the significance for their 'view of the world', it is important to stick with the principle you preach for: not to rely 'on the dubious value of...summaries instead of on original sources' (Martin 1986, p.421).

For example, Whorf (1940) mentions 'snow' in the Eskimo languages not to provide an extensive analysis of this particular language but rather to illustrate the point that different languages classify things differently:

> Whorf shows that the Aztecs represent 'cold', 'ice', and 'snow' by the same basic word with different terminations; 'ice' is the noun form; 'cold', the adjective form and for 'snow', 'ice mist'. Though not so radical, in English we 'have the same word for [1] falling snow, [2] snow on the ground, [3] snow packed hard like ice, [4] slushy snow, [5] wind-driven flying snow – whatever the situation may be. To an Eskimo, this all-inclusive word would be almost unthinkable; he would say that falling snow, slushy snow, and so on, are sensuously and operationally different, different things to contend with; he uses different words for them and other kinds of snow.' (Whorf 1956, p.216) [inserted numbers are mine].

Compare the interpretation and criticism of this single quote by prominent professional linguists, for example:

> [I]n his 1940 amateur linguistics article 'Science and linguistics'... Our word *snow* would seem too inclusive to an Eskimo, our man from the Hartford Fire Insurance Company confidently asserts... Notice That Whorf's statement has illicitly inflated Boas' four terms to at least seven (1: 'falling', 2: 'on the ground', 3: 'packed hard', 4: 'slushy', 5: 'flying', 6, 7, ...: 'and other kinds of snow'). Notice also that his claims about English speakers are false; I recall the stuff in question being called *snow* when fluffy and white, *slush* when partly melted, *sleet* when falling in half-melted state, and a *blizzard* when pelting down hard enough to make driving dangerous. Whorf's remark about his own speech community is no more reliable than his glib generalization about what things are 'sensuously and operationally different to the generic Eskimo.' (Pullum 1991, p.163).

Martin (1986) and Pullum (1991) emphasize that it is impossible to calculate the exact number of words for 'snow' in the Eskimo language family because these languages contain a great deal of grammatical endings and word formations. To follow these critics' advice not to rely on hearsay or amateurs' conclusions, it is only logical to consult a professional who knows the subject under discussion, in the form of Lawrence Kaplan (2003), Professor of Linguistics specializing in the Inupiaq Eskimo language, compiling dictionaries of Inupiaq and working on texts and grammatical explanations for the language. In his analysis, he is meticulous up to the smallest detail, for example: '[Whorf] clearly suggests that Eskimo languages have *five* or more snow words' (Kaplan 2003; emphasis is mine). Professor Kaplan provides a thorough analysis of the articles in question:

Treatment of actual data is ancillary to Martin's primary purpose of demonstrating the careless handling which the snow example has received... She reports that 'There seems no reason to posit more than two distinct *roots* that can be properly said to refer to snow itself (and not, for example, to drifts, ice, storms, or moisture) in any Eskimo language. In West Greenlandic, these roots are *qanik* "snow in the air; snowflake" and *aput* "snow (on the ground)". Other varieties have cognate forms. Thus, Eskimo has about as much differentiation as English does for "snow" at the monolexemic level snow and flake...' Martin does not handle the data particularly well, taking snow terms in West Greenlandic to be representative of those found in all Eskimo languages. The Comparative Eskimo Dictionary lists three... noun stems which would fit her criteria of referring to 'snow itself' and not to other related atmospheric phenomena... Another problem between Martin's equation of the two West Greenlandic stems meaning 'snow' with two English words is the inclusion of 'flake' as a basic English snow term. While 'flake' often refers to snow, it is generally used in conjunction with the word 'snow'... It may also be used with a variety of other meanings unrelated to snow, e.g., flake of paint... If we disqualify 'flake' that leaves 'snow' as the solitary English snow word (Martin's criteria), and Eskimo languages with three times that many! (Kaplan 2003).

Kaplan suggests we use the same (Martin's) criteria in relation to 'sleet, slush, blizzard' and other terms that do not include the word snow. If they had been included then we should have included the Inupiaq terms that denote some type of snow. The specialist's conclusion is very clear: Inupiaq has an extensive vocabulary for snow and ice. 'A minor quibble with Pullum is that he calls the bungling treatment of the snow example a hoax, even though there was never really any intention to deceive... Linguists and others familiar with these languages have always taken it for granted that there is extensive vocabulary for the areas in question' (Kaplan 2003).

13. For more information about autistic (non-verbal) languages see Bogdashina 2004.

14. Whorf emphasizes the importance of the theory of linguistic relativity for the development of science – no individual is free to describe nature with absolute impartiality because of the restrictions imposed by certain modes of interpretation.

15. However, we have to bear in mind that qualitative differences in experiencing sensations and interpreting the outside world vary for different individuals.

16. However, some argue that it is not necessarily the case and often refer to Stephen Wiltshire, a talented autistic artist. Like Nadia's, Stephen's language development was delayed. Though Stephen showed his drawing abilities

later than Nadia (who started at the age of three), at the age of seven, he still had no language when his talent first appeared. Unlike Nadia, Stephen's skills did not decline when he started talking at the age of nine. However, unlike Nadia, Stephen was intensively coached by a professional art teacher, so the continuation of his ability after the emergence of language can be seen as the replacement of 'savant skills' with those of a trained artist (Humphrey 1998).

17. For critical analysis and refutation of this assumption see Daria 2008.

18. The two main brain areas associated with language have been known as Wernicke's and Broca's. Wernicke's area is believed to be responsible for speech comprehension, and Broca's area for speech production.

NON-VERBAL COMMUNICATION 7

Some autistic individuals rely on intuition much more than on what is available on the surface. In this context we have to discuss non-verbal communication and the alleged difficulties or impairments with it which are attributed to individuals with autism.

The importance of non-verbal communication is undeniable. According to Alton Barbour, author of *Louder than Words: Non-verbal Communication* (1976), verbal communication comprises only a tiny part of social interaction. Communication can be roughly divided into:

- verbal (using words) – 7%
- vocal (using rhythm, intonation and volume, etc.) – 38%
- facial expression and body language (posture, gestures, etc.) – 55%

One of the defining aspects of autism spectrum disorders (ASDs) is said to be individuals' difficulty communicating both verbally and non-verbally. While that might be true about verbal communication for those individuals who do not understand speech (for example, because of their auditory processing problems), or are too literal in their receptive and expressive language, (paradoxically) many autistic individuals are (much) better in receiving non-verbal communication than their non-autistic communicative partners. I have to explain that here I do *not* mean traditional understanding of non-verbal communication, that is, a combination of body language, posture, facial expressions, gestures, and so forth. In this case, people with autism do experience difficulties and might be confused by conventional means of non-verbal communication.

Some researchers believe that ASDs are primarily a disorder of non-verbal communication (Tantam 1988, 2009). Non-verbal communication is often divided into two types: (1) a signalling system, and (2) subliminal communication (e.g. Tantam 2009). Signalling function is expressed by gestures, facial expressions and body postures that convey a message, for instance, lifted eyebrow can be read as 'Oh, what a surprise, I didn't expect that'. This and other signals are social; 'normal' people learn them from a very early age and become very skilful at sending and receiving them, without too much thinking. The signal type of non-verbal communication is similar to verbal communication – we send and receive messages that are understood by others of the same culture because they are culturally specific and learnt expressions.[1]

Some gestures are part and parcel of speech; they do not disappear even when a person talks on the phone and the listener cannot see him (Alibali, Heath and Myers 2001). Such gestures seem to help the speaker to talk and are reported to be absent in autistic children (Mitchell *et al.* 2006).[2] Some researchers (Ekman and Friesen 1972) distinguish other types of gestures as well:

- *Emblems* (learnt gestures): These may substitute as signs for verbal language in certain situations; for example, at a meeting when it is impractical (and rude) to talk aloud to your partner while listening to the presentation, or when hearing is impaired.

- *Illustrators*: These are culturally specific and are used to emphasize what one is speaking about, for example, an outstretched palm being turned up to indicate that the speaker does not know what is going on.

The second type – subliminal non-verbal communication – refers to the ability to read very subtle cues of social behaviours and adjust your own behaviour accordingly (Loveland 1991); for instance, to lower your voice when you want to say something about the person who is present in the same room, but you do not want him to know that you are talking about him, or to move and return a gaze to show understanding of a social situation. This type of non-verbal communication is even more difficult for persons with autism to understand.

The information conveyed non-verbally is mostly automatic. We do not consciously think, for example, 'I don't like this person, his presence makes me uncomfortable, I'll express it with my posture' or 'I'm so happy to see him, so I have to put a smile on my face and make a welcoming gesture'.[3] Professor Tantam (2009) has coined a new term – the 'interbrain' – to define a specific sort of automatic, nonintentional 'connectedness' through non-verbal communication, normal for neurotypicals, while those with ASDs are cut off from other people (being 'socially offline') because they have impairments in conventional non-verbal communication. From early age neurotypical children become:

> ...connected to each other and to their parents and other adults via the interbrain... [T]hey are therefore constantly attuning to and being influenced by communication with the parent. Some knowledge can be acquired...without the child even being aware of it happening. (Tantam 2009, pp.110–111)

Let us look at being 'socially offline' or 'disconnected from interbrain' from the perspective of differences in sensory perceptual processing. Those who experience a great difficulty in filtering out irrelevant (from the point of view of 'normal' people) sensory information and for whom sensory overload is the result of any attempt to socially connect with or understand people would inevitably struggle to 'connect':

> ...my hearing began to intensify as I headed for self-initiated sensory torture at the hands of my friends *because* I was

curious enough and interested enough to tune in… This was the price I was meant to pay…

I was sick to death of my attention wandering onto the reflection of every element of light and color, the tracing of every patterned shape, and the vibration of noise as it bounced off the walls. I used to love it. It had always come to rescue me and take me away from an incomprehensible world, where once having given up fighting for meaning, my senses would stop torturing me as they climb down from overload to an entertaining, secure, and hypnotic level of hyper…

The people-world was showing me a world I couldn't have…[and] it was not closed out by choice but by disposition. I was driven to want it like someone who finds her true home but finds she's been locked out. (Williams 1999b, pp.112–113)

With all these very real difficulties, starting very early in life, how could autistic babies socially connect to those around them? It is only logical that their non-verbal conventional communication becomes impaired and they fail to connect to others via the interbrain.

However, if we examine the behaviours that typically go under 'subliminal non-verbal communication' more carefully we can see that they apply to social responses, that is the behaviours we have *learned* to use in interaction with others (that have become automatic) rather than subliminal non-verbal communication *per se* (interpreting the term 'subliminal' literally as: 'below the threshold of sensation or consciousness'). The examples above (like lowering your voice to prevent someone hearing what you say) are not subconscious (though they may be automatic); they are learned behaviours. It would be more precise if we identify subliminal signals (non-verbal communication proper) as the signals that go unnoticed by the majority because their expression is involuntary and below the threshold that 'normal' sensory systems can detect.

The social world of the interpretive being may involve utilising a learned interaction system involving what is known as (interpretive) 'language' and (interpretive) 'manners'.

The social world of sensory being may involve using a learned interaction system involving what is known as (sensory-based) 'language' whether physically based or non-physically based. The sensory being may use sensory-based (non-mental) empathy through resonance in a relationship between sender and receiver in which the receiver loses their own separateness in merging with the sender as part of the mechanism of acquaintance before returning to the unmerged state of its own entity. (Williams 1998, p.117)

So, if we move away from 'traditional abilities' to interpret non-verbal clues we are supposed to pick up while communicating with someone, we have to admit that there is much more to non-verbal signals than just what we see and how we can interpret it. Besides, if someone is lying they try to control their body language, facial expressions, tone of voice and so on in order not to expose the lie, which makes it even more difficult to see through deception.

It turns out that many non-autistic individuals are not skilled in non-verbal communication (proper), either – they miss the 'leakage' of non-verbal information that is sent unconsciously (Ekman and Friesen 1969). In many cases, our facial expressions, postures, gestures, vocal intonation and so forth are non-conscious: we do not notice what 'messages' we are sending. The majority would not notice such subtle non-verbal clues as the way they sit or stand, how they look at someone, how they shape their mouths, and even the smell they give off, and will take what they are told on the surface level. Some individuals have developed the skills to interpret these 'messages' and trained themselves to become 'mind-readers', magicians or even 'psychics'.[4] They learn how to 'tune in' to their environment.

Some autistic individuals seem to achieve the same skill without training. Many of them (especially when they are young) interpret everything by intuition, by a 'system of sensing' (Williams 1998).

> I could tell from the change in the pattern of a footstep or the slightest change in the sound of the vehicle pulling up outside the feel of the occurrences about to happen. I could tell in the shifting pattern of movements, from strong to erratic, to flowing, to extreme, the range of possibilities that would follow. I could tell from the sound with which a glass was put down, in response to the sound of another glass being put down, the basic feel or 'edges' of the interaction that would take place. I could tell from the incongruence between what was being portrayed and what I could sense, whether chaos was impending or fear and reactiveness in the air... I wasn't 'psychic' in the common media sense of the word. It was merely that my system was quicker, less mechanical, less plodding than the system of interpretation. (Williams 1998, p.46)

> Being able to know what people are up to also is the cause of my indecision. It is like receiving multiple signals at the same time, because most things involve more than one person. It is my theory that most of the ability to predict human behavior depends on pattern-recognition skills which occur intuitively. (Schoonmaker 2008)

> Non-verbal people are masters at reading slight differences in a teacher's or parent's actions. I had one parent tell me their child has ESP because he is already waiting at the door *before* his mother even gets her car keys or purse. It is likely that the individual is sensing slight differences in behavior before it's time to get the keys or purse. There may be some hustle and bustle activities such as throwing out the newspaper... [T]he child may be responding to the sound of the paper being crushed in the trash can. (Grandin 2008, p.90)

Autistic individuals (especially those at the so-called non-verbal, low-functioning end of the spectrum who rely on their system of sensing) are more aware of the details that average 'normal' people have been missing. These individuals get much more accurate non-verbal information than others, because they 'tune in' their environment and listen to the intuition, and not to the intellect that might 'interpret' the opposite to the way they 'feel'. They use what Donna Williams calls 'the system of sensing' as opposed to conventional verbal and non-verbal interpretation.

> Having lost sensing, most people use the 'appear' as foreground information. To the sensory being, the 'be' is the foreground regardless to the degree to which one is socially trained and pressured to respond to the 'appear' as though, falsely, it was the 'be'. I used to go around unable to perceive the 'appear' because it was so background that only the 'be' stood out. (Williams 1998, p.111)

Such individuals can be easily overwhelmed by (and, sometimes, terrified of) the signals and stimuli 'normal' people are 'emitting' (and are unaware of), for example:

> Whatever the reason, I felt instantly unwell and sometimes terrified if I were face-to-face with a person, or even a thing like a wall or a chair...because I had too much impact from the complexity of depth, movement, colour and smell from any human being. (Blackman 2001, p.28)

We send out more information than we realize. Many animals and some people can 'read' these messages, because they are 'written' in non-verbal languages. The essence of any communication is to transmit or receive a representation of an experience. Representations restricted to verbal mode alone might be too feeble to excite by resonance, thus giving a very approximate description of the experience. Non-verbal communication proper (typical for animals, for example) may be a rediscovery in the deep unconscious of the pre-linguistic modes which are the natural modes of the mental field (Sheldrake *et al.* 2005).

Individuals with autism are known to experience difficulties to express their emotions both verbally and non-verbally and pick up these subtle cues as they are a part of social interaction. The clinical studies of people with ASDs reveal that it is their spontaneous facial expressions that are inhibited or impaired while they have no problems with producing voluntary facial expressions (Tantam 2009). The experiments show that people respond to emotional expressions unconsciously, and emotions seem to be contagious (Hatfield, Cacioppo and Rapson 1994); people involuntary mimic facial expressions of those with whom they interact (Surakka and Hietanen 1998). It can explain empathy when people 'feel' others' moods (Sonnby-Borgström 2002). 'Emotional contagion' develops very early in life and by the age of two years is fully established (Hay 1994). There is some evidence that the perception of someone's facial expression activates the neurons that would produce the same expression in the self (Preston and de Waal 2002). This is interpreted as proof of the existence of mirror neurons[5] and that suggests the sense of intersubjectivity (Trevarthen and Aitken 2001) that is closely connected to the development of empathy. When people pose a facial expression in response to a smile, for example, they begin to experience the emotion that goes with it (Tantam 2009). Tantam (2009) suggests that individuals with ASDs do not show this involuntary response; this, in turn, may lead to a lack of empathy, or they simply do not recognize the 'conventional expression of emotions'.

An adult with autism, Jim Sinclair wrote a very insightful article on this topic. He argues that no one ever bothered to explain to him that they expected to *see* feelings on his face, or that it confused them when Jim used words without corresponding expressions. When Jim was 25, with the help of his friend, he was able to learn to talk about emotions and with some effort to recognize them in others' facial expressions (Sinclair 1992). Marcie Kimball, a person with an ASD (2005), considers emotions as non-verbal communications disconnected from speech and language:

Autistics may not be consciously aware that they have perceived emotion because it cannot register while the brain is busy understanding what someone else is saying and while constructing what to say next. If the person is projecting a complex emotion, the autistic may perceive that something is going on but he/she doesn't know what it is. Occasionally, in true confusion, I've asked others if they are serious about what they have just said or, in other circumstances, 'Why are you looking at me like that?' More often, I've come away from a conversation, only to realize later that someone was 'making a face' that was supposed to indicate something. Many times, even after excessive rumination, I can't work out what it indicated because I don't have enough experience with that particular person to come to a conclusion. (Kimball 2005, p.20)

Some autistic individuals state that they can read the emotions of others more accurately when they can observe them without having to think in language (Kimball 2005), that is, in situations not 'clouded' by language. Another interesting idea expressed by some high-functioning autistic individuals is that people with autism have their own means of non-verbal communication and find it much easier to understand and empathize with other autistic people who do share many similarities in the ways that they move, behave and react to the world, which often makes sense to others with ASD even though they may be utterly confused with anyone else (Kimball 2005; Williams 1998).

Despite having difficulties identifying (conventional) emotional cues that are easily 'read' by 'normal' people, some autistic individuals are very hypersensitive to the emotions of others, which can sometimes becomes mixed with their own emotions that they can not easily separate them. Stephen Shore (an adult with Asperger syndrome) calls this phenomenon 'echoemotica', or taking on other people's moods and emotions and not being able to separate them from their own:

> This happens with most people to some extent, and quite often in children who pick up on a parent's or a teacher's emotion and act out accordingly. At this point in my life though I know that if I feel an emotion that's out of context with the environment, I need to look around and say, for example, to my wife, 'Are you feeling upset or agitated today?' Once I find out that she does feel upset, I can then separate from her feelings, still empathize with her, but also realize that it's not my emotion. In doing so, I've cognitively built typical empathy. (Shore 2003, p.90)

Temple Grandin reflects on her childhood memories of wanting to be hugged but experiencing panic because the emotional sensation was so strong and powerful that her involuntary reaction was to pull away; the sensation was too overwhelming as though a tidal wave was drowning her. Being touched by another person was so intense it was intolerable (Grandin and Johnson 2005). Autistic individuals who are 'emotionally hypersensitive' may experience 'emotional overload'.

> Raised in the Episcopal church, I was once removed from my pew, at age six, because I could not control my weeping. Unbeknownst to anyone, I had been staring at a terrible, glorious stained-glass window of the crucifixion and grieving for the pain Christ must have endured. The arresting mosaic of the forlorn image etched itself indelibly upon me. (Stillman 2006, p.4)

Even if emotions are positive, autistic tolerance of the 'emotional expression' of others can be very low. A 'language filter' protects verbal thinkers from the very powerful and vivid images experienced by autistic individuals (Daria 2008). A brain imaging study by UCLA psychologists has revealed that verbalizing our feelings and labelling our emotions make our sadness, anger and pain less. When volunteers were shown pictures of angry fearful faces there was an increased activity in the amygdala, that served as an alarm to activate a cascade of biological systems to protect the body in times of danger; but when the picture was accompanied with the label of the emotion shown, the amygdala was less active (Lieberman *et al.* 2007).

Tantam hypothesizes that lack of empathy in autism can be explained by lacking connection to the interbrain, because empathy requires the capacity for emotional contagion, or connection to the interbrain, 'so that we are provided with information about what another person is thinking, through their gaze, and feeling, through mirroring their facial expressions or some other means of emotional contagion' (Tantam 2009). If this is true, how can we explain the ability of some autistic individuals to be in resonance with other people? For example:

> It is rare that I know what anyone is actually thinking, but concurrent emotions are very common. (McKean 1994)

> 'I can walk into a room and feel what everyone is feeling,' Kamila Markram says. 'The problem is that it all comes in faster than I can process it. There are those who say autistic people don't feel enough. We're saying exactly the opposite: They feel too much.' (Szalavitz 2009)

The explanation might be in 'getting information' via different channels, rather than through conventional ones (gaze, facial expressions, etc.). Thus, contrary to present stereotypes, they can experience strong positive 'emotional connectedness' with objects, animals and people. Some autistic individuals 'sense' people and their inner emotions despite their communicative partners' attempt to hide them (Williams 1998).

> Autistics are acutely aware of emotional projection, due to not being able to filter out sensory input and mono-processing of emotions, even if they cannot identify the exact emotion that is projected (when the emotion is more complex)... The emotional mode can be one of merging with one's environment to the point where one feels as if he/she mixes with other people, animals, and objects. (Kimball 2005, p.25)

> I physically felt the pain when someone banged themselves. Around someone with a broken leg, I felt the pain in my leg. (Williams 1998, p.59)

Sometimes these and similar experiences are dismissed as 'new agey'. However, there is a growing body of research that confirms that these experiences are real for some individuals and are reflected in the activity in certain regions of the brain. For example, recent research has shown that some individuals find it difficult to distinguish between touch sensation caused by observation of someone being touched and by physical touch (Banissy and Ward 2007; Blakemore *et al.* 2005); some experience real pain when observing another person in pain (Jackson *et al.* 2006; Bufalari *et al.* 2007). These and similar studies confirm that at least some people have an actual physical reaction while observing others being injured. Dr Stuart Derbyshire and colleagues (University of Birmingham) have conducted a functional magnetic resonance imaging (fMRI) study to record the brain activity of people observing noxious events. The researchers have found that that some reported an actual noxious somatic experience in response to observing another person in pain. These individuals ('responders') comprise one third of the sample. The study shows that while observing images or video clips of someone in pain, the 'responders' show activity not only in the emotional centres of the brain (as 'non-responders' do) but also a greater activity in somatic brain regions (Osborn and Derbyshire 2010). These findings provide convincing evidence that some people can experience both emotional and sensory components of pain while observing others' pain, resulting in a shared pain experience.

Despite difficulties in (conventionally) 'connecting' to other people some autistic individuals 'feel' people instinctively or intuitively. Donna Williams describes how she feels or knows people by their 'edges' – 'the "be" beyond "appear"…the truth beyond the façade'. She says that 'they are the essence beyond the overlay of acquired constructed pseudo-personality' and 'the foundation of selfhood; its body without clothes that either fit it or disguise it' (Williams 1998, p.68). She describes this phenomenon in more detail here:

> Fluffy edged people...had a presence that was bubbly and warm...were emotionally expressive...seemed to drift or bounce along...
>
> Hard edged people, by contrast, had reins on emotion. They took control of it...
>
> Sharp edged people were unpredictable, their patterns often chaotic, staccato in their expression. These were reactive people...ruled by...constructed-false self, rather than the logical-practical-decisive mind...
>
> Crisp edged people...appeared strong but it was more that they 'held themselves' together than that they possessed a true solidness of self...
>
> Brittle edged people were those who had been fluffy edged people who had become damaged by life in some way. Brittle edged people were breakable, sometimes resulting in a mild defensive reactiveness but more often resulting in turning inwards...
>
> Sometimes people were generally entirely one type of edge or another regardless of who they were with. Others changed from one type to another depending on company. (Williams 1998, pp.66–67)

Some people with ASDs have reported they 'feel' other people's attitude towards them,[6] for example:

> I know when people do not like me, or find me strange and scary, no matter how polite and friendly they try to look. I just *physically* feel their attitude to me... I cannot describe it in words, it's just a 'feeling' that manifests through physical reaction in my body. I just sense someone's negative attitude, it may be quite painful... Strangely enough, even positive emotions towards me are felt as uncomfortable (though different from the negative ones) if they are too strong: they

engulf me... Both scenarios may result in panic. (P. T. 2002, personal communication)

[B]ecause autistic people perceive sensory phenomena in detail, the resulting emotional impact on them can be compounded. Many must find ways to shield themselves from emotional onslaught. This is even more exaggerated due to the simplicity of emotions that are evoked. Rather than experience various emotional blends, they may just get irritated by another who is being somewhat emotionally negative. (Kimball 2005, p.19)

For those who rely on the system of sensing (Williams 1998) it is extremely hard to understand that others are unable to do it and rely mostly on what they see:

In a world which has learned to rely on the system of interpretation and either to deny or make redundant the system of sensing, it is unnaturally *natural* that people should have an unspoken consensus not to look beyond the surface and to believe and trust and live by the experience that what they see on the surface is all that there is. It is, perhaps, equally unnaturally natural that such people may be at once curious and threatened by challenging encounters with those for whom this is not their assumed reality. (Williams 1998, p.87)

From this perspective, we can see that it is 'normal' people who are disconnected ('off-line') from 'sensory-emotional feel' typical for highly sensitive autistic individuals:

To my horror, when challenged to drop these facades, I found people defending them fiercely as though these were their 'real' selves. They took it further, considering my response to them weird and finally, when enough people had had similar responses, I eventually assumed they must have been right. I must have been broken, deeply deluded, on the wrong planet. The thought that most people had cancer of the soul or had bought into a sort of social mass psychosis they called 'normality' was just a symptom of how crazy I'd actually become. (Williams 1998, p.86)

Is it any wonder that not many individuals have come out with their 'weird' experiences? The prospect of being considered 'crazy', 'psychotic' or 'psychic' is not very appealing. However, many parents do believe that their children are able to feel their emotional states, but, for the same reason, they are afraid to articulate their suspicions. For instance:

My daughter is ten and she has autism. There have been many times throughout her life when I wondered if she is clairvoyant or can read minds. There have been times when I have been thinking a question and she has answered it verbally. There have been times when the phone or doorbell rung and she said the person's name that was there (relatives she knew). (Stillman 2006, p.153)

Quite a few adults with autism confirm that such experiences are real, for example:

...I saw the milkman approaching me. Instantly, I knew what he wanted. Again, there was no explanation for how I could possibly know. I never before realized how often I do this, because it is so automatic and I used to habitually ignore it. I can't control the ability to know what people are up to. It is something that happens *to* me. It's not something I can make happen whenever I want. (Schoonmaker 2008)

Donna Williams describes similar occurrences in *Autism and Sensing*.

It has been claimed by some carers and professionals using Facilitated Communication (FC)[7] with disabled (including autistic) people that their clients display telepathic abilities; for instance, one professional reported how '[a] mother said that her adult son has no need to hear what she and his other two facilitators want him to know: he simply types his responses to their unspoken comments' (cited in Haskew and Donnellan 1993, p.14).

Even many proponents of FC try to avoid the 'offending term', though, and find a more rational explanation for incidents of seeming telepathy, as 'cueing' (whether conscious or unconscious). Thus, the originator of the technique of FC, Rosemary Crossley (1993), discounts the reports that the facilitated are reading the facilitators' thoughts and states that the most likely explanation for any incident of 'telepathy' is cueing, whether conscious or unconscious, sought or unsought. Professor Biklen (1992) accepts the idea that a facilitator (subconsciously) gives cues to the facilitated, thus influencing their messages. Ann Donnellan suggests that possibly the facilitated learns to 'read' the facilitator in some subliminal way (cited in Sitzman 1998). In their book *Emotional Maturity and Well-Being: Psychological Lessons of Facilitated Communication* (1993), Haskew and Donnellan put forward a possible explanation of why there are so many reports of telepathy among those who have (mental) disabilities in contrast to 'normal' people whose telepathic abilities are usually elusive:

> It may be that a sixth sense is present in all of us at birth, but as speech and locomotion develop, the need for it fades. Still, many people seem to retain vestigial psychic abilities, especially at times of accident or trauma, and there is much anecdotal scientific literature describing those. For people with impaired communication capabilities the sixth sense may remain active and utilized. The speaking world is simply rediscovering it. (Haskew and Donnellan 1993, p.9)

Kristie Jordi, the author of *A Child of Eternity* states that only about 10 per cent of their respondents experience some kind of unusual phenomenon (for example, 'reading minds') with their autistic or otherwise disabled child or student (cited in Sitzman 1998).[8] If only we could accept that some people perceive, interpret and communicate differently, and did not deny them the right to use the systems they are comfortable with, while helping them adjust to the world around them, both sides would have won:

> Those who appear not to seek to make sense of their environment may not necessarily be 'retarded', disturbed, crazy or sensorily impaired, but may, in spite of not using the same system everyone else uses, still have one of their own. They may, in spite of apparent delayed development, actually continue to use a system that others have left behind very much earlier. (Williams 1998, p.53)

The danger of this approach lies, of course, in the conventional negative attitude to the phenomena we cannot explain; for instance, the above examples are interpreted as telepathy and the official position towards it is non-acceptance. However, we can look at this phenomenon from a different perspective – as a form of non-verbal communication. Professor Josephson believes his research may provide an explanation for paranormal 'spookiness'. If electrons can jump around the lab instantaneously, then surely it might be possible for one brain to tell another what it is seeing without using normal methods of communication? Freud defined telepathy as a primitive form of communication made dormant by language; in other words, it is the ability mentally to communicate thoughts, emotions, words or images silently to another person (Stillman 2006). Stillman compares it to meditation or prayer when people send spiritual communications to the Higher Power.

We can get a better understanding of 'non-verbal communication proper' if we study animals' communication, most of which is non-verbal. They do produce sounds or 'words' but only to warn about danger, attract a mate, frighten an enemy, or when in pain. However, animals' primary communication is non-verbal. Those who live with humans communicate 'verbally' only when addressing their owners – a cat asking us to open the door, for example. (You would not see two cats sitting and meowing to each other about their plans for the day.) Most of the time they communicate non-verbally, or we may say 'telepathically'.[9]

There is nothing mystical or supernatural in animals' 'telepathy'. For instance:

1. In some cases, it is the sense of smell (undetectable by humans) that animals use to 'read' messages about the health of their owners (for example, dogs detecting cancer in humans, or oncoming seizures). Another example is that of Oscar, the cat who seemed to sense approaching death of people in the care-home. Animals can smell fear as well.

2. Given that animals do not develop verbal language, they are more 'open' to receive non-verbal information. Often it is their ability to interpret 'invisible' cues humans and other animals send out. The 'Clever Hans' story,[10] often used to refute animal intelligence, illustrates, in fact, animals' unique ability to 'read' humans' unconscious body language, movements and facial expressions.

3. Animals have the ability to 'read' patterns of sounds or movements, providing them with information about, for instance, the emotional state of someone.

Often humans communicate to animals unintentionally and then are surprised how their pets know that they are taking them to the vet or going on holiday. While animals pick up messages, humans call them 'psychic'. But there is nothing psychic about their ability to 'read' or pick up messages – they have been doing it all their lives.

An animal communicator, Carol Gurney, explores the ways humans can learn to communicate with animals in her book *The Language of Animals: 7 Steps to Communicating with Animals* (2001). Gurney insists that animal communication is neither new nor controversial. The question is not 'When did we begin to be able to communicate with other species?' but 'When did we stop?' According to Gurney, the main factor in animal communication is the ability to listen, which means to become tuned or more sensitive; and it is possible to learn how to use our intuition, to allow ourselves to really feel as the animal feels.[11] This ability is natural to young children, but as we grow older (and become intellectually oriented) this ability is suppressed. Intuition is like a muscle that needs exercise (Gurney 2001). Another interesting observation is that animals are very much a reflection of us. They reflect (resonate with) our emotions and inner feelings (Gurney 2001). Often humans just do not 'listen to' them; they ignore the messages their pets are sending them. That is why many of the pets have learned to communicate to their owners by other means – for example, dogs bringing their lead when they want to go for a walk.

Some autistic individuals are said to have a special connection with animals. This issue has been investigated by Temple Grandin in her acclaimed co-authored book *Animals in Translation: Using the Mysteries of Autism to Decode Animal Behavior* (Grandin and Johnson 2005). As people with autism are mostly perceptual thinkers,[12] it is no wonder that some of them can understand the non-verbal behaviours of animals. Grandin speculates that:

> Autistic people's frontal lobes almost never work as well as normal people's do, so our brain function ends up being somewhere in between human and animal. We use our animal brains more than normal people do, because we have to. We don't have a choice. *Autistic people are closer to animals than normal people are.* (Grandin and Johnson 2005, p.57)

Rupert Isaacson, a father of a boy with autism, writes about the special relationship that his young son Rowan developed with Betsy, a horse:

> Without hesitation, Rowan opened his arms and hugged Betsy's great brown head, which was hanging low enough for him to reach. Then he gave her a kiss. As he did so, an expression of extraordinary gentleness came over her – a certain softening of the eye, a blissful half-closing of the eyelid with its long black lashes. Something passed between them, some directness of communication that I, a neurotypical human, could never experience. (Isaacson 2009, p.34)

We may assume that non-verbal individuals who do not develop understanding of verbal language might, instead, develop other ways to interpret information intuitively, and what we call 'telepathy' can be one of these ways. The problem is, however, how can these children know that others are unable to do it?

Developing his hypothesis of the interbrain, Professor Tantam (2009) explores the idea of connection not only between people but also people and nature:

> The intuition that there is another side of human experience, in which we are cells in a super-organism rather than self-determining individuals, has repeatedly surfaced in philosophy and literature. During the European enlightenment the bee hive was often taken as an analogy of the state, and the interconnectedness of citizens whose individuality was less important than their labour. In the last century bee hives and ant societies have been routinely considered by biologists to be super-organisms and individual bees themselves as super-cells within that organism. (Tantam 2009, pp.101–102)

Tantam illustrates his idea about connectedness with examples from group therapy (where group therapists sometimes feel as if the individuals in the group have fused together into a matrix, in which ideas and emotions circulate and resonate like signals between transistors in a radio) and links it to a number of theoretical perspectives, namely 'intersubjectivity' and Jung's 'archetypes'.

While individuals with ASDs can be *socially* offline (Tantam 2009) they still can have much deeper subconscious emotional connections with people with whom they have a very strong bond. Carers often report that their children or clients feel calm if they themselves are calm, and agitated if the carer feels nervous (Tantam 2009). Working with families with autistic children I have met mothers who confided that they believed their offspring can 'read their emotional states' even when there are miles between them. (Unfortunately, but understandably, very few of them are prepared to talk about it publicly.)

I've always known that my son reacts to my emotional states and I do my best to compose myself and 'feel good' when we are together, but now I suspect that even when I'm far away our special emotional connection is always there.

Last November, I had to go abroad for a very important meeting [connected to her job]. I left everything prepared for my 18-year-old autistic son who was staying with his relatives (it had worked many times before). When I arrived to my point of destination very late at night, I was terrified to find out that nobody was there to meet me (as was previously agreed). So, there was I, late at night, in the airport in a foreign country with no money, no address of the hotel, and no language... I panicked...

Eventually, I managed to phone to my friend in England who found the contact's phone number in the country I was in, and arranged someone to come and pick me up from the airport. I stayed there for three days, in a very bad mood, which I couldn't get rid of. I remember thinking, *It's good that my son is not with me, or he would be unmanageable.* Little did I know – he *was* unmanageable but...back at home. When I returned and saw the damage he'd done to the house and bruises he inflicted to the people he loved, the only explanation we could find was his reaction to my disaster far away. (Mrs. C. 2008, personal communication)

The notion of connectedness is acknowledged in quantum mechanics. For example, such quantum theorists as d'Espagnat and David Bohm argue that we must accept that, literally, everything is connected to everything else: 'We may safely say that non-separability is now one of the most certain general concepts in physics' (d'Espagnat 1973, p.734).

Each and every particle seems to 'know' what other particles are doing and reacts accordingly. The Aspect experiment (designed to detect the two photons emitted together from one source to fly apart and to measure their polarizations) shows that the measurement made on one photon simultaneously affects the nature of the other. This and similar experiments have proved that some interaction links the two particles, even if they are moving apart at the speed of light. These findings provide us with a very different world view from our everyday common sense interpretation:

> They tell us that particles that were once together in an interaction remain in some sense parts of a single system, which responds together to further interactions with other particles right back through time... We are as much parts of a single system as the two photons flying out of the heart of the Aspect experiment. (Gribbin 1991, p.229)

Bergson hypothesized that people are far less definitely cut off from each other, soul from soul, than they are body from body:

> It is by their bodies that the different human personalities are radically distinct. But if it is demonstrated that human consciousness is partially independent of the human brain, since the cerebral life represents only a small part of mental life, it is very possible that the separation between the various human consciousnesses or souls, may not be so radical as it seems to be. (Bergson, cited in Gunn 1920)

He suggests that in a physical world there may be a process analogous to what is known in the physical world as *endosmosis*.[13] Bergson suggested that it was probable, or at least possible, that a subtle and subconscious influence of soul to soul was constantly taking place, that was unnoticeable by active consciousness. The philosopher argued that we have no right to deny its possibility just because it is considered to be 'supernatural':

> for our ignorance does not entitle us to say what may be natural or not. If telepathy does not square at all well

with our preconceived notions, it may be more true that our preconceived notions are false than that telepathy is fictitious... We must overcome this prejudice and seek to make others set it aside. Telepathy and sub-conscious mental life combine to make us realize the wonder of the soul. It is not spatial, it is spiritual. (Bergson, cited in Gunn 1920)

Stillman provides a very interesting argument:

Children and animals, as purest of innocents, often perceive spiritual experiences only because they haven't yet been conditioned *not to*... The person with autism may simply not be fully cognizant of her very special gift, and may assume that *everyone* communicates in this way. (Stillman 2006, p.70)

Donna Williams (1998) offers her explanation of the phenomenon: the body is more than a physical form; it is also an energy form. Some people's energy boundaries are more 'open' than most people's. These are the individuals most prone to a wider range of 'psychic' experiences and 'déjà vu'. This state is involuntary, beyond their control. They can either give in to it or try to fight it.

In the 1960s a Czech psychologist, Milan Ryzl, investigated the mental power of two supposedly telepathic people who were many miles apart (Ryzl 1966). The 'sender' was told to try to make the 'receiver' uncomfortable by imagining that he had been buried alive; as a result, the 'receiver' experienced an attack of asthma. Ryzl's experiments were inspired by the theory of his colleague Stepan Figar who had proved that when one person concentrates on another, it can cause a measurable rise in blood pressure. Figar's theory was confirmed by the experiments conducted by Professor Douglas Dean (Dean and Nash 1963). In similar experiments conducted by Dr Stefan Schmidt and colleagues (2004) at the University of Freiburg, Germany, the electrodes attached to the receiver's skin registered 'prickling' sensations in the skin.

These and similar experiments show that the 'telepathic feeling' seems to depend on emotional bonds – the stronger the emotional bond between two people, the stronger the feeling (and success rate) of 'telepathy' is. There is a similarity with 'animal telepathy' between social animals (who live in packs, herds, flocks, etc.) A communicable sense of danger keeps them together and helps them survive predators.

A very interesting phenomenon – 'distant touching' (touching with the eyes) – has been reported in autism. Some individuals experience being touched when someone is looking directly at them; these sensations may make them feel very uncomfortable: 'Eyes are very intense and show emotions. It can feel creepy to be searched with the eyes' (O'Neill 1999, p.26).

A mother of an autistic child has found that she does not have to tell her son to stop doing something (when he misbehaves) or shout to attract his attention; just staring at him brings the desirable results – 'Don't look! I won't do it again, I promise.'

This can be a form of synaesthesia that produces physical sensations without the individual being physically touched; for example, looking at something can feel like touching it:

> The only animals I enjoyed watching [in the zoo] were the seals. Because they were like a tactile experience for the brain. (Blackman 2001, p.65)

> I have a synesthesia thing where color and touch were crossed. (Williams 2007)

Or, some autistic individuals experience 'being touched' by sounds:

> [S]ometimes I had a crossover effect where real sound flashed through my brain from what my eyes picked up and what my skin had sensed... Hearing certain sounds gave me more of a skin- than a brain response. Extraordinarily some sounds are still processed in both areas, and others only involve what I call 'sound-feeling'. 'Sound-feeling' may come from sounds other people cannot hear. (Blackman 2001, pp.18–19)

We can see some similarities between autistic individuals who rely on the system of sensing (and in many cases, are non-verbal) and shamans. The ability to understand 'non-verbal communication proper' ('telepathy') seems to be present at the very dawn of civilization and it seems to have taken humans thousands of years to get rid of it. The earliest example known to us is a shaman.[14]

McKenna describes the shaman of the past as a kind of sanctioned psychotic who was able to move into states of mind so extreme that his immediate social efficacy was arguable; just by perturbing the ordinary brain states and ordinary language states shamans were able to reach hyper-dimensional understanding. It is said that shamans can talk to animals. McKenna speculates that behind shamanism is the idea that human and animal consciousness can be very closely intertwined, and that early humans may have been telepathic like, and with, their animals (McKenna in Sheldrake *et al.* 2005).

The psychological state of shamans has been a dominant preoccupation of multidisciplinary work on shamanism since the beginning of the last century. While some scholars (Boyer 1962, 1964, 1969; Handelman 1967; Noll 1983) believe that shamans have no mental problems, others insist that shamanic behaviour was and is the result of a mental disorder (Bogoras 1907; Czaplika 1914; Devereux 1961; Silverman 1967). Some scholars (Bourguignon 1976; Lex 1979; Noll 1983; Siikala 1978) argue that the shifts in psychological states of shamans are within the boundaries of normal behaviours. It seems, with time, that the description of shamanic states has been moved from the category of abnormal psychology to the category of universal psychobiological capacities (Atkinson 1992). However, psychological abnormalities in connection with shamanism are still occasionally mentioned in scholarly literature. Since the 1960s there has been a shift in thought to identify shamanism with altered states of consciousness to such an extent that these two terms are sometimes used as interchangeable.[15]

As shifts in consciousness are a key part of shamanic practice (Atkinson 1992), there have been attempts to clarify what is distinctive about shamanic states of consciousness, though no consensus has been achieved. Walsh's study (1989) offers a 'phenomenological mapping' of different states of consciousness, including shamanism, schizophrenia, Buddhism and yoga. The researcher indicates that there is a variety of psychological states with considerable differences among them. While some scholars (for example Peters and Price-Williams 1980) define shamanic ecstasy as a particular form of altered state of consciousness, others (Winkelman 1986) argue that the shamanic trance state is not unique and is found in all kinds of magico-religious practitioners. Still others (Goodman 1990) go even further and insist that there is one religious or ritual state of consciousness comparable with a Chomskian deep structure that underlies surface differences in the experience of this state.

A very interesting model of the interactions among shaman, spirits and patients that leads to altered states of consciousness was put forward by Siikala (1978). Recognizing a great diversity of shamanic traditions, Siikala's model still offers possible ways to identify common features among them. She argues that 'the technique of communication used by the shaman as a creator of a state of interaction between this world and the other world is fundamentally an ecstatic role-taking technique' (p.28). According to Siikala, the psychic process of this shamanic technique is the same as the technique used in hypnosis. Noll (1985) argues, however, that the achievement of an altered state of consciousness is a means to promote enhanced mental imagery.

If we put aside social and cultural dimensions of shamanism and focus on the psychological characteristics, the most important and overriding feature of shamanism is thought to be the state of consciousness shamans achieve during shamanic practices (Benarik, Lewis-Williams and Dowson 1990). Ridington (1990) cites a definition that identifies shamanism as 'an institutionalization of a transformation from the ordinary waking phase to a nonordinary one, in which internally generated information comes to dominate and override decision-making and orientation function of the waking phase' (p.125).

A very interesting analysis of the products of shamanic altered states of consciousness is provided in the work of Lewis-Williams and colleagues (Lewis-Williams 1987; Lewis-Williams and Dowson 1988). These researchers studied the rock paintings of Southern Africa, the Great Basin and Upper Paleolithic Europe as illustrations of the shamans' altered states of consciousness.

Of particular interest are the interpretations of the cave paintings, dating to about 30,000 years ago, which were discovered in Chauvet at the end of the last century. The majority of scholars interpreted them as clear evidence that their makers must have possessed high-level conceptual thought. In contrast to these claims, in his article 'Cave art, autism, and the evolution of the human mind' (1998), Nicholas Humphrey put forward the idea that drawings on the walls of the Chauvet cave were made by humans with pre-modern minds who had little symbolic thought and no interest in communication. Humphrey came to these (controversial) conclusions after having compared the cave drawings of animals with drawings made by Nadia, a non-verbal autistic savant, who at the age of three showed an extraordinary drawing ability – line-drawings of animals with a photographic accuracy and graphic fluency – but who had no language at the time and no ability to think conceptually. Humphrey provides a list of remarkable similarities between the cave paintings and Nadia's sketches, such as the striking naturalism and realism of the individual animals (in contrast to our 'normal' stereotyped images-concepts of different classes of animals); the similar graphic techniques used to achieve the drawings and the tendency for one figure to be drawn on top of another (Humphrey 1998). He suggests that drawings of this quality are never produced by untrained artists *unless* they are autistic.

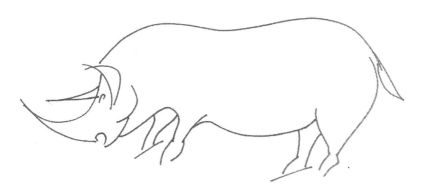

The engraving of a rhinoceros in the Chauvet Cave

Originally, the researcher assumed that the cave art indicated the pre-conceptual and pre-linguistic mind of the humans 30,000 years ago. After the publication of 'Shamanism and cognitive evolution' by Michael Winkelman, who hypothesizes that 'cave art images represent shamantic activities and altered states of consciousness, and the subterranean rock art sites were used for shamanic vision questing' (p.7), Humphrey introduced certain corrections to his original idea. In his 'Commentary on Michael Winkelman'. Humphrey avoids putting things as a simple 'either-or antithesis' but rather poses a question – What if shamans resembled autistic savants *some of the time*?

> Deep within the caves, suffused with music and dance, inspired by whatever constituted their ice-age soma, their memories primed, their senses sharpened, regressing to the state of 'innocent perception' of which Huxley speaks. Perhaps it was in that state that they were able to recall in quasi-photographic detail the sightings of wild animals; in that state that they were able to trace the outlines of these images as if projected by a lantern onto the cave wall. (Humphrey 2002, p.93)

That is, Humphrey is suggesting that they became *functionally autistic* (being *temporarily* in a non-conceptualizing state of mind) only during their 'activity of shamanizing' by entering an altered state of consciousness which suppresses conceptualization. The suggestive evidence for this possibility can be found in some of the literature on psychotic drugs, including Aldous Huxley's classic account of his experiments with mescalin (Humphrey 2002).

Notes

1. Some non-verbal signals may have different meanings in different cultures; for example, in Bulgarian society nodding your head means 'no', while 'yes' is expressed by shaking the head.

2. However, those autistic individuals who 'speak kinaesthetic' seem to use gestures that help them 'shape their thoughts' into verbal speech (for more information see Bogdashina 2004).

3. Darwin (1872) argued that facial expressions in humans evolved from movements indicating intentions to communicate, which he called an intention movement; for example, when someone wants to comment he or she opens their mouth. Such movements eventually evolved into a system of communication.

4. For example, Marc Salem, a psychologist, has been interested in exploring the mind and its potential. He has been working in several universities studying and lecturing psychology, especially the development and nature of mental processes, with a speciality in non-verbal communication (www. marcsalem.com/about.cfm). Salem has mastered his amazing ability to unlock hidden mental powers and become a very successful entertainer, who has performed his show 'Mind Games' around the world. He gives seminars to corporate executives on improving their memory skills and interpreting non-verbal signals from business opponents, trains lawyers on how to choose jury members and teaches communications at college. Salem calls himself a 'mentalist', or, sometimes, a 'thought reader'. According to him, a thought can be guided, because the mind is shifting and changing every second (Witchel 1997).

   Derren Brown is a psychological illusionist, well-known for his 'mind-reading' skills that allow him to predict and control human behaviour. His television and stage performances have entranced millions. Brown describes some of his 'tricks' and methods in his very readable book *Tricks of the Mind* (2006).

5. Diaccomo Rizzollati conducted experiments on monkeys, recording signals from parts of the frontal lobes which are concerned with motor commands. The researcher found that there are cells that fire not only when the monkey performs certain specific movements but also when the monkey watches another monkey performing the same action. Rizzollati terms these neurons mirror neurons ('monkey-see monkey-do neurons'). It has been suggested that mirror neurons are dysfunctional in autism (Dapretto *et al.* 2006; Hadjikhani *et al.* 2007; Lee *et al.* 2006). Professor Tantam (2009) remains sceptical about the role of mirror neurons in ASD and cites studies to show that the evidence is inconclusive: there are research findings for an impaired ability to imitate (Smith and Bryson 2007) but also for an unimpaired ability (Bird *et al.* 2007) and some evidence that mirror neurons are intact in autism (Hamilton, Brindley and Frith 2007). In fact, autistic individuals may be very good imitators. For some, it is vital to see other people doing certain activities in order to be able to perform these activities, for example:

> As usual I used my companion (in this case my mother) as if she were a reflection of myself. This assured me that what I understood my body to be doing was exactly what it was doing, just as I liked to be sure that I was an actual part of the person whom I was using to model my own existence, by insisting that the other person and I performed similar actions. This occasionally appeared in every day life by my either eating or drinking to catch up exactly with the other person or, more inconveniently, by my insisting that he or she emptied her glass or cleared his plate to exactly the same point that I had reached if I were ahead. It was only by seeing what I had done actually happen that I could be sure that I was doing. (Blackman 2001, pp.233–234)

Besides, many people with an ASD are excellent mimics – able to take another person's way of speaking, moving, etc. (Tantam 2009) in order to disguise their difficulties in understanding social and communicative conventions (Bogdashina 2004), for example:

> I had been…able to mimic sound or movement without any thought whatsoever about what was heard or seen. Like someone sleep-walking and sleep-talking, I imitated the sounds and movements of others – an involuntary compulsive impressionist. This meant that I could go forward as a patchwork façade condemned to live life as a 'the world' caricature. (Williams 1999c, p.9)

> [When all else failed] I used to rely on a 'fitting in' trick that is nothing more than a sophisticated form of echolalia. like a professional mimic I could catch someone else's personality as easily as other people catch a cold. I did this by surveying the group of people I was with, then consciously identifying the person I was most taken in by. (Willey 1999, p.57)

Sometimes I feel like my interactions with the environment involve many little pieces of other personalities I come in contact with. These little bits get compressed and employed here and there. (Shore 2003, p.90)

6. A typical response to this is 'As one of the classic features of Asperger syndrome is the inability to read emotions and empathize, and so on, [they] appear to be in the minority in knowing "when people don't like me".' Yet again, I have to remind the reader that not *all* autistic individuals experience these states, but it is not the reason to deny this ability to those who do. As for 'the classic features' – difficulties with or inability to read emotions, empathize, and so forth, they can be interpreted differently if we look at them from the 'autistic perspective'. For a detailed discussion, see Bogdashina 2005.

7. Facilitated Communication (FC) is a type of augmentative and alternative communication for people who do not speak or whose speech is highly limited and disordered and who cannot point reliably (Biklen 1990; Crossley 1992). FC is a very controversial method that has brought a huge amount of both positive and negative responses in the field of autism. It is not the aim of this book to provide a discussion of all the pros and cons of this method (For a review, see, for example, Bogdashina 2004, pp.235–243; success stories – www.inclusioninstitutes.org/fci; stance taken by various agencies on FC – www.religioustolerance.org/fc_comm4.htm).

8. Judith Netzer-Pinnick summarizes astounding conclusions by some proponents of FC:

   [T]he surprising fact [is] that the less literate the subject, the more articulate are the communications. On the premise that the phenomenal world, of which literacy and verbal communication are a part, is less real than the unknown world in which mental communications originate, it is not illogical that the less there is of this real dimension, the less it will interfere with the communication. (Netzer-Pinnick 1998)

9. A possible explanation of animals' 'telepathic abilities' has been suggested by Rupert Sheldrake (1999, 2004) who investigated hundreds of cases of dogs and cats who can 'predict' their owner's behaviour long before the human displays it. In his book *Dogs that Know When Their Owners Are Coming Home* (1999), Sheldrake provides his survey of over 1000 randomly chosen pet owners who reported 'strange' abilities of their pets, such as knowing that their owners are about to go on holiday before they have even started packing, or when they are about to be taken to the vet. Sheldrake believes that the 'unusual abilities' displayed by animals are, in fact, manifestations of a single capacity (a 'morphic field') to be very sensitive to changes in the activities, emotions and intentions of people.

10. In the beginning of the twentieth century, a retired German maths teacher discovered what he thought to be amazing capabilities and human-like intelligence in his horse Hans. The horse seemed to know many facts from different disciplines and could answer questions by tapping his foot an appropriate number of times. However, a psychologist Oscar Pfungst, who was sent to investigate Hans' superabilities, found that the horse was unable to answer any question if the person posing a question did not know the right answer, or stood behind the screen and Hans could not see him. Pfungst concluded that Clever Hans was using very subtle visual cues to get his answers right.

11. However, it is important to distinguish between those individuals who can 'feel' animals' emotions or exchange mental imagery, and those who claim to get 'verbal messages'; the latter are likely to be frauds.

12. Not all of them are necessarily 'visual'.

13. *Endosmosis* – the inward flow of a fluid through a permeable membrane toward a fluid of greater concentration. In osmosis (the movement of water molecules from an area of high concentration to an area of low concentration), it is the more rapid spread of the less dense fluid through the membrane to join the more dense. Cell membranes are completely permeable to water, therefore, the environment the cell is exposed to can have a dramatic effect on the cell.

14. Here we will focus on the study of shamanism as an example of different states of consciousness. For a review of the development and analysis of multidisciplinary research on shamanism see Atkinson (1992).

15. Some shamanic traditions (such as 'psychedelic' shamanism) are connected to using hallucinogens in order to experience visions and sensations during shamanic seances (Browman and Schwartz 1979; Dobkin di Rios and Winkelman 1989; Furst 1972; Harner 1973; Joralemon 1984; Wilbert 1987).

SENSORY HYPER-SENSITIVITIES 8

Autism sensitivities seem to be caused by a kind of cleansed perception unrestricted by language. Sometimes they can be seen as extrasensory perception (ESP) as those around them not only fail to see, hear, smell or feel what some autistic individuals can, but also find it hard to imagine that these experiences are possible. Let us look at the most common features of 'autistic perception' that can shed some light on the possibility of the 'unusual experiences', bearing in mind that qualitative differences in experiencing certain stimuli are different for different individuals. Hypersensitivities to sensory stimuli are very common in autism. The senses of some autistic individuals may be too acute and they may see, hear, feel, and so on stimuli that are undetectable by 'normal' people. For instance, William Stillman writes about some individuals with autism who even react to positive ion changes in weather systems (Stillman 2006). Jasmine O'Neill feels that it is her autism that enables her to experience her surroundings in a very intense way, both physically and emotionally. She describes her senses of hearing and smell to be so finely tuned to the environment that she reacts to tiny changes in weather patterns and atmosphere pressure the way an animal would (O'Neill 2003). Tito could actually feel the energy and *see* its pathway:

> The intensity of the energy in [the] room was very strong. I felt like a small raft floating in the midst of [it]. The energy bounced across the room, all around the walls, the pictures reflected them, and the tables diverted them toward the ceiling... I could actually see the pathway of the energy wave, bouncing around with speed. (Mukhopadhyay 2008, p.196)

Examples of seeing colours while hearing sounds in synaesthesia are well known. Some individuals seem to see not only the colours of their acoustic environment but also the density, shape and movement of sounds. For example,

> I could hear nothing but social talk from voices, which slowly formed a collective tunnel around me. I could gradually see the tunnel turning solid around me, as more voices gathered to shape it. Its opaqueness prevented me from seeing the wall or the ceiling or the bouncing energy across the room that I had seen before. I saw myself in that tunnel, within its diameter. (Mukopadhyay 2008, pp.196–197)

While 'crossing the tunnel' in order to 'see the light and breathe in fresh air' (p.197), Tito actually crossed the street to come to the door of the house opposite. His mother followed him, and it was her voice that melted the tunnel back into the conventional physical world. Tito emphasized that it was not sleepwalking because he was very aware of what he was experiencing and the experience was so very real he could replay it any time. Trying to understand this phenomenon, Tito looked for clues in texts on neuroscience and came up with his own explanation of what had happened and why: all experiences are broken into several components (language units, belief units and emotion units, and units of action) and stored in the mind. The same experience may be stored and interpreted by different persons in different ways, depending on how their units are stimulated:

> As my mind goes beyond the physical definition of light and air, I can easily transfer my thoughts to some other observation, far from the physical interpretation. So it is very natural for me to feel that the air from the table fan is trying to blow away some of the intensity of the light from the surface of this page. Although it is not physically happening, it is the story my mind has formed. (Mukhopadhyay 2008, pp.198–199)

Barsalou (1999) emphasizes that perceptual symbols are multi-dimensional, originating in all modes of perceived experience, and are distributed widely throughout the modality-specific areas in the brain. This researcher considers the perceptual aspect in a wider sense: rather than just referring to the sensory modalities, it refers to any aspect of perceived experience.

Research findings confirm what individuals with autism have been saying and writing about for decades. For example, the Ashwin *et al.* (2009) study has revealed that the autistic group exhibited visual 'acuity so superior that it lies in the region reported for birds of prey' (p.17). Another recent study has shown that children with autism performed better than normally developing children on difficult visual search tasks (O'Riordan *et al.* 2001). Increased sensitivity to vibration was reported by Cascio *et al.* (2008) and enhanced auditory discrimination by O'Riordan and Passetti (2006). It has been suggested that autistic brains are 'tuned' to higher frequencies (Blakemore *et al.* 2006) possibly due to neuronal micro-architecture (Casanova, Buxhoeveden and Gomez 2003).

This 'higher-vibration' capacity of the senses goes parallel with the acute, often overwhelming sensitivities to sensory stimuli, when certain stimuli (which are different for different people) are very disturbing to individuals with autism. For example, Temple Grandin (1996b) describes her hearing as having a sound amplifier set on maximum loudness. Some autistic individuals may be able to hear some frequencies that only animals normally hear. Others can see air particles that become a background with the rest of the environment fading away (Williams 1999b). Wendy Lawson describes how 'Noises seemed so much louder for me, and I had to move away from conversations at times because the noise hurt my ears' (Lawson 1998, p.30).

On the other hand, however, autistic individuals with their heightened senses can often appreciate colour, sound, texture, smell and taste to a higher degree than people around them (Lawson 1998). Here are some autistic individual examples:

While walking home from class I noticed a tiny, red insect covered in black dots crawling inside one of the hedges. I was fascinated by it, so sat down on the pavement and watched it closely as it climbed over and under the sides of each small leaf and branch, stopping and starting and stopping again at various points along its journey. Its small back was round and shiny and I counted dots over and over…at the time I did not think of anything but the ladybird in front of me. (Tammet 2006, p.70)

I find it perfectly exciting to study a nectarine growing on the tree in my garden. The smooth almost-round shape covered in red, orange and yellow with a green splash in the middle is most exhilarating! To be able to watch them grow and develop is a miracle that never ceases to amaze me. To take half an hour to look at one does not seem strange to me – indeed it is hard to take my eyes away from the fruit even after such a length of time. I could never understand the apparent apathy of my friends to the rich intensity and feelings in colours. I could tell they were not impressed by my 'finds'. (Lawson 1998, p.4)

Fascination with sensory stimuli is quite common in autism. Sometimes people with autism, when they have given up fighting in an incomprehensible world, rescue themselves from overload by escaping to an entertaining, secure and hypnotic level of hyper-sensation: watching the reflection of every element of light and colour, tracing every patterned shape and vibration of noise as it bounces off the walls (Williams 1999c). Donna Williams names it as the beautiful side of autism, the sanctuary of the prison. Autistic individuals can be fascinated with different sensory stimuli, such as the smell of melting candles, rice cooking, the feel of velvet or marble, the taste of smooth, satiny wood, the pit-pat of bare feet on tiles, the look of clouds gliding high, the feel of a horse's nose, the chalky taste of seashells (O'Neill 1999). The sources of fascination are very individual. For example, to some people certain visual patterns are appealing; others may find certain colours fascinating. A typical picture of an individual with autism is when he is sitting staring transfixed at a crystal, turning it around and around in front of his eyes, catching rainbows (Williams 1999c). In this sense, autistic perception can be seen as superior to that of so-called normal people. They are 'shaken out of the ruts of ordinary perception' (Huxley 1954/2004, p.46).[1]

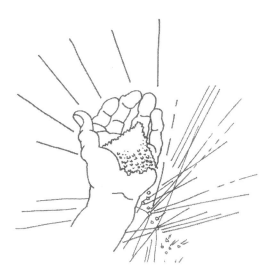

It is also interesting to compare Huxley's description with those of some individuals with autism:

I looked at a film of sand I had picked up on my hand, when I suddenly saw the exquisite beauty of every little grain of it; instead of being dull, I saw that each particle was made up on a perfect geometrical pattern, with sharp angles, from each of which a brilliant shaft of light was reflected, while each tiny crystal shone like a rainbow... The rays crossed and recrossed, making exquisite patterns of such beauty that they left me breathless... Then, suddenly, my consciousness was lighted up from within and I saw in a vivid way how the whole universe was made up of particles of material which, no matter how dull and lifeless they might seem, were nevertheless filled with this intense and vital beauty. For a second or two the whole world appeared as a blaze of glory. (Huxley 1956/2004, p.62)

When left alone, I would often space out and become hypnotized. I could sit for hours on the beach watching sand dribbling through my fingers. I'd study each individual grain of sand as it flowed between my fingers. Each grain was different, and I was like a scientist studying the grains under a microscope. As I scrutinized their shapes and contours, I went into a trance which cut me off from the sights and sounds around me. (Grandin 1996a, p.44)

The nursery was my first experience of the outside world and my own recollections of that time are few but strong, like narrow shards of light piercing through the fog of time. There was the sandpit in which I spent long periods of the day picking and pulling at the sand, fascinated by the individual grains. Then came an obsession with hourglasses...and I remember watching the trickling flow of sand over and over again, oblivious to the children playing around me. (Tammet 2006, p.21)

However, there may be negative side-effects to this fascination: it is like an addictive drug; the more you do it, the more you want to do it (Grandin 2008). The longer someone stays in this state, the more addictive it becomes, and the person may miss out on

developing social skills and experiencing the life of the majority
(e.g. Mukhopadhyay 2008; Williams 1998).

Note

1. One can find many similar descriptions in the literature of religious
   mysticism and in poetry.

SIDE-NOTES: BEFORE WE GO FURTHER

9

People with autism and other developmental disabilities have been looked at with either fear or awe, and other emotions in between. Seeing autism as something to be feared of (or wondered at) is quite understandable when the nature of the condition is as yet not fully known. The less we understand, the more we fear; and fear rarely (if ever) brings positive reactions. For example, some children with autism have been seen as possessed by an evil spirit; desperate parents, influenced by some good-intended but ill-informed church authorities, have even agreed to exorcism as the only option to free their child from a supposed evil spirit. Some tragic incidents have been reported in the newspapers where children were restrained and suffocated during an exorcism ceremony.[1]

Other parents go to another extreme and try to find favourable explanations that border on mystical interpretation, for instance, calling children with autism crystal or indigo children, crediting them with supernatural abilities or connections to angels. The New Age approach, though popular, seems to be an area where speculation is not balanced by an appropriate amount of scepticism (Sheldrake *et al.* 2005).

Where are we now?

The attitude of the official scientific community is so opposed to anything conceived as supernatural that those who genuinely try to understand these (not necessarily supernatural, but yet unexplained) phenomena are afraid to speak out. For example, Donnellan, who wrote about facilitated communication (FC) with autistic individuals, seemed to be afraid even to mention telepathy in her article and felt it necessary to emphasize that she just reported experiences which others had claimed happened, rather than her opinion, in fear of being discredited. Yet even her carefully chosen words and disclaimers did not protect her from critics (Dr Spitz) who discredited her work anyway (Sitzman Undated). Treffert, a leading specialist in autistic savants, received some angry 'how dare you' letters to the editor saying that he was compromising his scientific integrity by mentioning the possibility of extraordinary experiences, when he 'dared' only report that it had been reported! (Autism AWARES On-Line Conference, December 2007) Not very well understood phenomena, like telepathy, supernatural abilities, déjà vu and other so-called (but not necessary) 'psychic' experiences are very difficult for outsiders to identify. Bill Stillman (2006, p.11) writes about quite a few adults with autism who prefer to remain silent about their experiences in order not to risk 'antagonising others' perceptions by fuelling stereotypes of "autistic behaviour", only to be explained away as delusions or psychotic episodes and medicated accordingly'.

However, many parents do feel that their children are able to read their minds (not to be confused with the Theory of Mind),[2] but they are afraid to articulate their suspicions for the same reason.

Samuel (2009) points out that science progresses as much through the selective use of evidence to support particular scientific models and frameworks as through the objective and impartial evaluation of alternative modes of explanation. The researcher emphasizes that the point is not that the particular models and frameworks endorsed by current scientific thinking in any specific field are mistaken but rather that alternative approaches have been excluded, 'on the assumption that there can be only one truth, and that if one model is successful all other models are valueless' (Samuel 2009, p.90). For example, many possible healing techniques have been routinely dismissed because they cannot be evaluated through canonical methods of the contemporary biomedicine (see, e.g. Adams 2002; Kaptchuk 1998). Samuel argues that it is not science, but 'scientism' – 'the naïve belief in the absolute priority of a particular kind of scientific research'. This suggests that a dismissal of other explanations as scientifically illegitimate may be 'missing something vital' (*Ibid*.). As Clarke (2000) puts it, if we do not understand a certain phenomenon, it does *not* prove that it can never be explained, but merely that at this stage of our ignorance it is far beyond the scope of today's science.

> There is no such thing as the paranormal and the supernatural; there is only the normal and the natural and mysteries we have yet to explain. (Shermer 2006, p.38)

In comparison with exact sciences (mathematics, physics, etc.) psychology seems to be a cinderella as within the field 'knowledge to mystery must be the smallest of all' (Maslow 1970, p.46). Because there is so much to know in comparison with what we do know, Maslow puts forward the definition of a psychologist, 'not as one who knows the answers, but rather as one who struggles with the questions' (Maslow 1970, p.46).

If we feel so uncomfortable with discredited labels (and want to distance ourselves from distortions and sort out the wheat from the chaff), maybe we could change the 'names' we use for these phenomena. There have been precedents we can relate to: to avoid mentioning 'offensive' terms some researchers introduced euphemisms, such as, for example, 'exceptional situational awareness' used to describe the performance of some jet fighter pilots who respond faster than they 'should' be able to in combat dog-fights (Hartman and Secrist 1991). Other terms include 'anticipatory systems', used to describe how biological systems plan and carry out future behaviour (Rosen 1985), and various terms like 'postdiction' (Eagleman and Sejnowski 2000), 'subjective antedating' (Wolf 1998), 'tape delay' (Dennett 1992) and 'referral backwards in time' (Libet 1985) – all referring to neurological mechanisms proposed to explain how sometimes we are conscious now of events that actually occurred in the past (Radin 2000, p.12). The change in the labels we apply will allow a more open approach to research, observation and interpretation. For instance, as we have seen, one of the participants at the Autism On-Line Conference (2007) suggested the term 'prospective intuition' to describe the ability to anticipate events before they have happened.

If we replace special psychic abilities and channelling or receiving messages from other worlds with 'sensitivities to otherwise unnoticed sensory stimuli (due to differences in brain functioning) of the same physical world' in the following sentence, maybe it would make us look at the phenomena differently, with an open mind?

'Some people with autism possess *special psychic abilities* to receive messages *from other worlds*.'

'Corrected' statement:

'Some people with autism seem to be able to perceive the same physical environment with heightened sensitivity that allows them to see what others with "normal" sensory and cognitive functioning fail to notice.'

We do not deny animals' 'supernatural abilities'. We do not call them psychic, though.

Despite being invisible, difficult to imagine or supernatural for the normal population, some issues are recognized by the majority of researchers:

- Some autistic individuals are able to perceive stimuli that others cannot. For example, a child might hear (and be disturbed by) the sound of a microwave oven working in the next room but one; or someone can see a 60-cycle flickering of fluorescent lights that makes the room pulsate on and off; or a person tries to escape from the room because he cannot tolerate the smell of certain perfumes. The list is endless.

- Autistic savants whose calculating, artistic talent, musical ability is well known and recognized – even if we cannot explain how they do it, we do not deny their abilities.

- Synaesthesia – it is difficult to imagine how sounds can be perceived as colours, for example; but it is recognized as a real condition.

So what is so different about so-called 'supernatural experiences'? It is healthy to be sceptical about these phenomena but instead of denying their existence, isn't it more wiser (and more scientific) to accept that if we cannot explain certain things it does not mean they do not exist, so we should try to find a possible explanation?

> If we don't know something, it's better to accept that it is 'unknown as yet' than dismiss it altogether – 'It doesn't exist because I don't know it.'

Our history shows that sometimes what was ridiculed (or even punished) in the past becomes obvious today. For example, a few centuries ago the earth was considered to be flat, and the sun obediently rotated around it. Those who dared disagree ended their lives in flames. It has been happening since ancient times – every new generation seems to find it so hard to let go of their beliefs and accept new knowledge. It is true especially about so-called mystical and supernatural experiences. Any attempt to investigate anything out of boundaries of proper or true science brings suspicion, dismissal, anger and...labelling. This description of the situation in the last century is still very pertinent today:

> In the currently fashionable picture of the universe there is no place for valid transcendental experience. Consequently those who have had what they regard as valid transcendental experiences are looked upon with suspicion, as being either lunatics or swindlers. To be a mystic or a visionary is no longer creditable. (Huxley 1956/2004, p.98)

Before scientists could explain certain 'laws' in nature, like, for instance, lightning or tornado, these phenomena still performed perfectly well and did not wait for people to understand what was going on.[3]

John Gribbin (1991) reflects on the ideas Eddington expressed in his book *The Philosophy of Physical Science* (1958), one of them being that what we perceive, what we 'learn' from experiments, is highly coloured by our expectations. Eddington provides a very powerful example to illustrate it. Suppose an artist is sure that the shape of a human head is 'hidden' in a block of a marble, and to prove it, he takes a hammer and chisel and chips away the waste to reveal the hidden head. Eddington draws parallels with the artist's 'discovery' of a head and Rutherford's discovery of the nucleus, Dirac's discovery of a positron...

> Is it possible that the nucleus, the positron and the neutrino did *not* exist until experimenters discovered the right sort of chisel with which to reveal their form?... [T]he interpretation in terms of particles is all in the mind, and may be no more than a consistent delusion. The equations tell us nothing about what the particles do when we do not look at them, and before Rutherford nobody ever looked at a nucleus, before Dirac nobody even imagined the existence of a positron. (Gribbin 1991, p.162)[4]

The situation in autism research is very illuminating.[5] Some researchers cannot inhibit their bias and seem to know the results well before they start their investigation. For example, consider a case when a researcher publicly announces that autistics have no problems, impairments or distortions in sensory perception, that they are not different from non-autistics in their sensitivities, but they are superior in their perception and their ability to process information, and then conducts a study to prove it. It could have been laughable if it had not been so dangerous. Or another quite common mistake in autism research – studies are conducted with five to eight persons with high-functioning autism and Asperger syndrome, and then the results are interpreted in term of autism in general. At best, these results are useless; at worst, they are misleading. Qualitative research (case studies) are very important as they may give us ideas of subgroups and differences of perceptual and cognitive features in different people with autism, but quick and unreliable overgeneralisations (so typical for some researchers) create misinterpretation of the condition.

There are at least two general sources of evidence for 'unusual experiences': anecdotes and validation in controlled experiments. From an anecdotal perspective, there is no doubt that these experiences exist. As for control experiments, it is more controversial. Some have been replicated (making it more difficult to deny the 'reality' of these experiences); while others have failed. 'Failures', however, do not necessarily mean that the phenomena do not exist. The very nature of certain phenomena makes them difficult to replicate.

- Not everyone has these abilities (or to the same degree).

- 'Average' does not mean 'average' when we group people for research ignoring existence of subgroups. For instance, if visual thinkers are grouped together with kinaesthetic, auditory or tactile thinkers and given tests to assess their visual functioning, the 'average' results will be levelled to 'normal' (hiding performance peaks in visual thinkers, and below average visual functioning in individuals with kinaesthetic, auditory or tactile dominance).[6]

If we group 'average' individuals to measure unusual phenomena, the results will be insignificant. The fact of the matter is, though *all* people can potentially possess unusual abilities, very few can actually demonstrate, experience or master them. How would we interpret the average results of controlled experiments, therefore? A good example to illustrate this point is provided by Ramachandran who suggests it is easy to show that nearly all of us are synaesthetes but we are in denial about it. In one of his 2003 Reith Lectures, Ramachandran asks his listeners to imagine two shapes: one of them is a shattered piece of glass with jagged edges, the other is like an amoeba with undulating curvy shapes. Then he gives two 'names' – a booba and a kiki – and asks which name describes each of the shapes.

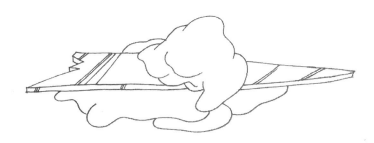

A booba and a kiki

Amazingly, 98 per cent of people will name the shattered piece of glass with the jagged edges as a kiki, and the undulating amoeboid shape as a booba, because, the researcher claims, we are all synaesthetes (Ramachandran 2003). Though we all possess the synaesthetic traits, comparatively very few individuals are at the top of the synaesthetic spectrum. The 'average result' would be meaningless.[7]

Research into sensory perceptual issues in autism is even more complicated. Sensory sensitivities and other differences in perception are very variable among individuals with autism, and often within one and the same individual. There are no two autistic individuals with exactly the same sensory perceptual profile (Bogdashina 2003). One person can have difficulty filtering visual information and be hypersensitive to visual and auditory stimuli while being hyposensitive in tactility and proprioception. The other might have normal vision but some difficulties in screening out auditory information and be hypersensitive to touch and smell. What complicates the matter even further is that one and the same individual may be hyper- and hyposensitive to the same stimuli, depending on the state of health, tiredness, stress and so on, because sensory perception can fluctuate in autism. As there are so many constantly shifting variables, it makes it difficult to design research studies to explore different unusual (often also called abnormal or bizarre) sensory experiences in autism. The same is true about designing studies to test therapies addressing sensory problems. For example, some professionals would insist that there is no research evidence that sensory integration therapy works with individuals with autism; there is no surprise here because of a huge variability of sensory problems in autism. We see a similar situation in research into other treatments, for example, special diets – lack of scientific evidence that diets work with individuals with autism is claimed despite numerous personal accounts that diets work. None of the approaches would benefit the average person with autism. Temple Grandin puts forward this argument: if 20 children are involved in the study and four benefit from the therapy, while 16 do not, is it ethical to deem the therapy ineffective? Even if the quality of life for these four children has improved tremendously? Don't they (and others like them) count? Surely, we must look at autism research from a different angle, for instance, posing questions like 'Why does...work for some and not for others?' Is it wise (and ethical) to overlook a large (and growing!) body of anecdotal support (Grandin 2008)?

How shall we interpret anecdotes? Shall we deny them as impossible (and/or irrelevant) or just a coincidence, or shall we study the phenomenon and work out methods to prove or dismiss it?

In the history of any science the collection of anecdotes preceded the analysis, formulation of hypotheses and experiments. The inevitable anecdotal evidence is necessary for research on such a heterogeneous subject as autism. If we accept that autism may be caused by different factors (i.e. we may assume there are 'autisms' that require a different approach in each individual case), then we have to accept that despite similar surface behaviours (known as the triad of impairments), certain subgroups can be singled out that would differ in their sensory perceptual, cognitive and linguistic profiles. It is qualitative research that can help to identify subgroups and bring understanding to certain sensory, cognitive, psychological and linguistic phenomena that go unnoticed in normal functioning.[8]

Notes

1. See, for example, Cohn, D. 'Autistic Boy Dies During Exorcism.' CBS News, 25 August 2003, www.cbsnews.com/stories/2003/08/25/national/main570077.shtml; Sweetingham, L. 'Exorcist's brother says God claimed autistic boy's life, not defendant.' CNN News, July 2004, www.CNN.com/2004/LAW/07/09/exorcism/index/html.

2. Theory of Mind (or 'mind-blindness') is defined as an inability to infer another person's mental states.

3. Arthur Clarke, who was seen as one of the great predictors of what was to come, wrote in the Introduction to the collection of his essays *Profiles of the Future: An Inquiry into the Limits of the Possible* (2000):

> With few exceptions, scientists seem to make rather poor prophets; this is rather surprising, for imagination is one of the first requirements of a good scientist. Yet, time and again, distinguished astronomers and physicists have made utter fools of themselves by declaring publicly that such-and-such a project was impossible... The great problem, it seems, is finding a single person who combines sound scientific knowledge

– or at least *feel* for science – with really flexible imagination. (Clarke 2000, p.6)

Clarke formulated three laws to be applied while contemplating what is impossible. The first law reads:

> When a distinguished but 'elderly' scientist states that something is possible, he is almost certainly right. When he states that something is impossible, he is probably wrong. (Clarke 2000, p.21)

Clarke provides plenty of examples to illustrate the foolishness of 'prominent experts'' analysis that has been proved wrong, with the development of science in different fields, who were ignorant enough successfully to 'forget' their own statements and jump to the bandwagon when the 'impossible' had turned out to become 'possible'.

Clarke notes that the first law was updated for political correctness in later additions (like the one the quote is taken from). Clarke explains his definition of the word 'elderly' in this law:

> In physics and mathematics it means over thirty; in other disciplines, senile decay is sometimes postponed to the forties. There are, of course, glorious exceptions; but as every researcher just out of college knows, scientists of over fifty are good for nothing but board meetings, and should at all costs be kept out of the laboratory. (Clarke 2000, p.21)

Strangely enough, these and similar views have been widely read, acknowledged and…ignored. Of course, researchers and scientists of today are more enlightened, progressive and know better of their field; what they need, however, is a good portion of scepticism directed to their own views and opinions.

4. It is telling that quite a few physicists have become interested in paranormal phenomena and defend their strong interest by pointing out that much of conventional modern physics is itself highly speculative. 'Some might say there is less evidence for superstrings than there is for ESP and at least we can try to replicate paranormal phenomena in the laboratory' (Carr 2000). Among them is the Nobel-prize-winning physicist Brian Josephson who is known for his pioneering theoretical work on superconductivity. Despite the mainstream (negative) attitude to the subject Josephson keeps investigating the brain and the paranormal. He believes that even if the phenomena may be difficult to reproduce, it does not mean the phenomena are not real.

   At present Josephson is the director of the 'Mind-matter unification project' at the Cavendish Laboratory, Cambridge.

   We still do not know much about how the universe works. Some scientists state that there are at least 11 dimensions – ten of space and one of time.

Although the extra seven (or even more) dimensions are invisible to us, they still manifest their existence as forces (Davis 1984).

5. Quite a few researchers have sprung out from nowhere to proclaim they are 'messiahs' bringing forth groundbreaking ideas. The problem with this approach is that those claiming to be pioneers in the field do not seem to know (or even want to know) that their groundbreaking discoveries were discovered many years ago. Their main arguments for claiming a pioneering approach seem to be: (1) neo-pioneers use different words to describe old concepts, for example, 'enhanced perception' to indicate 'oversensitivity'/ 'hypersensitivity'/'gestalt'/etc., and (2) the findings/ideas were not published 'scientifically' (i.e. they were in books but not in scientific journals). However, is everything 'published in peer reviewed journals' necessarily right? How can we interpret diametrically opposite results of scientific findings? For example, ask 100 people and 99 of them (including smokers) will tell you that smoking is bad for your health. However, while this seems to be true for lung diseases, the research (Ritz *et al.* 2007), published in the July issue of *Archives of Neurology*, based on the data of 11,809 individuals involved in 11 studies conducted between 1960 and 2004 suggests that smokers are less likely to develop Parkinson's disease. The sample is big enough to make the study's findings statistically significant. The authors found that smokers were less likely to get Parkinson's, and those who smoked more seemed to have greater protection. A potential explanation is the biochemistry of the brain. In Parkinson's, nerve cells – dopaminergic neurons – are lost in the part of the brain that controls movement. Dr Ritz, of the UCLA School of Public Health in Los Angeles, and her co-authors speculate that a substance in cigarette smoke may protect those nerve cells. Another research shows that coffee is a healthy drink that might actually reverse the effects of Alzheimer's. Dr Gary Arendash presented findings that caffeine can be a viable treatment for this devastating degenerative condition. Researchers at the Albert Einstein college of Medicine in New York published the results of a 13-year study (involving 7000 people) that shows that people who consume less than 6g of salt a day actually have a 'raised' risk of heart disease. And of course, there are studies that try to prove the opposite.

6. Dean Radin lists 8 reasons why replication is not easy:

(1) the phenomenon may not be replicable; (2) the written experimental procedures may be incomplete, or the skills needed to perform the replication may not be well understood; (3) the effect under study may change over time or react to the experimental procedure; (4) investigators may inadvertently affect the results of their experiments; (5) experiments sometimes fail for sociological reasons; (6) there are psychological reasons that prevent replications from being easy to conduct; (7) the

statistical aspects of replication are much more confusing than most people think; and (8) complications in experimental design affect some replications. (Radin 1998, p.40)

7. The test suggested by Ramachandran (2003) for ('above average') synaesthetes who see numbers as colours, for example, five as red and two as green, is as follows: researchers produce a computerized display on the screen with a random jumble of fives and embedded among these fives are a number of twos arranged to form a shape like a triangle or square. For non-synaesthetes, it takes as long as 20 or 30 seconds to see the shape formed by the twos, while the synaesthetes see it immediately.

8. Of course, it does not mean that we should believe all and every anecdotal claim. However, Carl Jung's warning is very relevant to the present state of affairs in the research of 'extraordinary' and 'unusual' phenomena. The statistical method aims to show facts in the light of the ideal average but does not give us a picture of their empirical reality. 'While reflecting an indisputable aspect of reality, it can falsify the actual truth in a most misleading way' (Jung 1958, p.5).

EXTRASENSORY REALITIES IN AUTISM (With Possible Explanations)

10

Extrasensory phenomena include (but are not limited to) so-called gut feeling or sixth sense, seeing or hearing what normal people do not see or hear, telepathy, premonition, déjà vu and so forth. Some of them have been moved from the supernatural category to the natural, while others are still awaiting understanding and explanation. Human senses and their functions are not as straightforward as they may seem. People are able to perceive far more than they can simply see, hear, touch, taste and smell. Ramachandran (2003) points out that our brains are capable of intersensory interaction – taking many different sensory inputs and combining them in unusual ways.

A sixth sense

There is no consensus about the phenomenon, nor about the name for it. Some people call it a 'sixth sense', others – 'seventh sense', still others – 'extra sense', or gut feeling. Whatever name you prefer, the phenomenon is defined as the ability to detect change or danger without conscious awareness, or a sensation of knowing something by instinct or intuition. This sixth or seventh sense seems to be more developed in some than others. Some people just feel that something is wrong; they seem to know what is going to happen. Until recently these (quite common) experiences have not been investigated scientifically, and have been dismissed as pure coincidence and superstition. However, in my view, there is nothing mystical about it.

According to a psychologist and computer scientist, Ronald Rensink (University of British Columbia, Canada), who has been researching this phenomenon, conscious mind is not the only thing dictating our perception and reaction; some decisions seem to come from parts of the brain not directly associated with conscious thought. An unconscious visual perception might be at work. His research suggests that people can be aware of – and can use – visual information without consciously seeing it because we have a distinct, fast-acting mode of visual perception that takes in visual information and makes us *sense* it, without consciously seeing it (Rensink 2004). This explains why people sometimes have an intuition or sixth sense about a situation before they can consciously understand what is going wrong or different. Rensink describes how 'humans appear to have a highly effective "pattern-matching" system that is unconscious but highly intelligent. These unconscious systems often communicate with the conscious mind by such gut feelings' (Rensink, cited in LaFee 2007).

'Seeing' can be defined as knowing by looking, that is, conscious visual experience. However, not all aspects of visual processing lead to visual experience (Rensink 2000b). In fact, quite a lot of experimental evidence (Merikle and Joordens 1997; Merikle and Reingold 1992; Milner and Goodale 1995; Schacter 1987; Weiskrantz 1996) indicates the presence of *sensing* – the processing of visual information without any conscious awareness. In addition to the research on blindsight mentioned in Chapter 5, evidence has been provided (e.g. Goodale 1993; Milner and Goodale 1995) that vision may consist of two largely independent systems: an 'on-line' stream dealing with immediate visuomotor action (for example, eye-movement, balance maintenance), and an 'off-line' stream dealing with longer processes, such as the conscious recognition of objects in the immediate environment. When the off-line stream is damaged (e.g. by a lesion), the person, while not consciously seeing and experiencing some part of the environment, is still able to interact with it in some way, for example pointing at or grasping the object.

As we have seen (in Chapter 2), change-detection experiments have shown that the visuomotor system responds to the change before there is conscious awareness of it. For instance, a subject is asked to grasp a rod, but the location of the rod is changed the moment the person tries to grab it. It turns out that an adjustment of the trajectory of the hand happens several hundred milliseconds before conscious report of the change (Castiello, Paulignan and Jeannerod 1991).

Rensink has empirically tested the ability to detect change or danger without conscious awareness of the individual in order to answer the question: can an observer consciously sense that a change is occurring but still have no visual experience of it? In one of his studies (Rensink 1998), 40 observers were presented with a flicker sequence in which a picture alternated with a similar one altered in some way. Observers pressed a button first when they were *aware* that something was changing, and then again when they *visually experienced* the change. Sensing was found to occur in a large number of trials. It is interesting that most of the successful trials were from a small number (14/40) of observers; half of the observers (20/40) experienced little or no sensing.[1] Rensink calls this phenomenon (an abstract mental experience without sensory experience) 'mindsight' (Rensink 1998) and suggests it may correspond to the 'sixth sense' (providing a warning to a person in dangerous situations). Rensink clarifies that mindsight is not only about vision but may be about other senses, too, for example, hearing – when you know someone is behind you, even when you cannot see them. The mechanisms underlying mindsight are not well understood yet, and the reason for the delay in conscious visual experience is unclear. Rensink speculates that the observer might have difficulty disengaging from the non-attentional mechanism, thereby slowing down the processes underlying the visual experience of change.

Another study, by Rollin McCraty, attempted to measure this elusive sixth or extra sense, or intuition. The volunteers were shown a series of images, most of them peaceful and calming, but they were interspersed with some shocking pictures of car crashes or snakes ready to strike. The volunteers' hands were connected to the machine that monitored their heartbeats and sweat secretion. Between five and seven seconds before they saw a shocking image the equipment showed increased heartbeat and sweating, indicating a subconscious fear response (McCraty 2004).

Joshua Brown, a researcher at Washington University, St. Louis and colleagues proposed a possible source for the feeling that something is wrong in the brain. They suggest that the anterior cingulate cortex (ACC), located near the top of the front lobes and along the walls dividing the left and right hemispheres, mediates between fact-based reasoning and emotional responses, such as love and fear. The researchers hypothesize that ACC works at a subconscious level and acts as a pre-emptive early warning system – to help us to anticipate the potential danger so that we can be more careful and avoid making mistakes. This region of the brain seems to monitor subtle changes in the environment, while leaving a person unaware of the process. This process takes place on a subconscious level, leaving us with an elusive 'gut feeling' we can not explain but we 'sense' that something is wrong. These 'feelings' are sometimes incorrect but they should not be disregarded altogether.

Other senses can be involved into ESP as well. It was thought that only animals could detect pheromones, but recent research has shown that humans can and do detect and react to pheromones released by others, even if they are not conscious of this. Researchers from Stone Brook University, New York (Mujica-Parodi *et al.* 2008) have conducted experiments that show that the sweat we produce when frightened is a signal that is subconsciously picked up by others.[2] A psychology professor Bettina Pause and colleagues at the University of Dusseldorf have conducted a research study revealing that the smell of fear not only exists but is easily catching (Pause *et al.* 2009). So emotions can be communicated chemically between humans. And it is not only fear that is coded in our body odour, we are constantly sending chemical signals that are (subconsciously) picked up by others.

There are numerous examples reported. For instance, Jim Corbett (2000) who spent most of his life hunting man-eating tigers in India described many an episode when his 'jungle sensitiveness' saved his life. His gut feeling made him cross the road to avoid a tiger. His unconscious mind directed his feet away from danger.

These strange powers exist in all people, but the majority do not seem to be tuned into them. However, in some individuals they are very much present, and in others they can reappear under certain circumstances.

Premonition or precognition

Let us look at what is known as premonition as a version of the sixth or seventh sense because it also involves detecting something that is likely to happen. In many cases, there is a very natural explanation to it. (In others, we may just not have discovered it yet.) For example, we are not surprised that many living organisms are able to predict changes in the weather. Many flowers, for instance, close their petals before the rain; swallows hunt low before bad weather; cattle will lie down in a dry spot before the storm. They feel changes in air pressure (nothing mystical about that). Animals are very skilled in predicting (sensing) disasters.[3] What is interesting is that animals can feel not only natural disasters but also man-made ones. Many cases have been documented when animals fore-warned their owners of explosions, road accidents, trees falling and so on. Does it mean they are psychic, or that they sense something most humans cannot? Is it a psychic or paranormal (out of this world) phenomenon or is it a perfectly natural ability possessed by some animals and some humans – to tune into something that scientists perhaps do not understand fully yet, which is quite natural and does not break any laws of nature? In some countries, where abnormal animal behaviour is taken seriously, human casualties have been prevented. For instance, in China in 1995 the city of Haicheng was evacuated early on the day of its earthquake because of widespread animal panic. The ability to sense danger or animal premonition has been reported by many pet owners. For example, dogs might refuse to go along the paths where, shortly afterwards, a road accident would happen (Sheldrake 1999).

Scientists have developed highly sophisticated equipment to detect shockwaves deep inside the earth to predict earthquakes before they happen. Even if normal people cannot feel these shockwaves, it does not mean they do not exist. Perhaps animals and some humans are able to detect them without any equipment because of their brains working differently.[4]

Some people have reported similar experiences, and, in my view, there is a great need to investigate the nature of them further.[5] To avoid the stigma attached to premonition or precognition, one of the participants of the online Autism conference has suggested changing the 'label' to 'prospective intuition'. Maybe then we can start afresh, without a biased attitude? We cannot explain these phenomena yet, but they do exist and are very real phenomena for those who have experienced them.[6]

Many examples of premonition (prospective intuition) can be found in personal accounts of individuals with autism and their parents. For example:

> There were odd occasions at school when I seemed to know things about people before they did. One day when two children were skipping rope and the game was getting intense, I knew that one child would fall down – I had hardly

seen the thought when it happened. I know this could easily be coincidence, but it happened many times. Sometimes I would dream of a place, in great detail, and then experience that very place at some future time.

In many ways, I felt my sensory perception was superior to that of my peers. I had the ability to hear noise before they did, which meant that I could tell when the school bus was approaching before others could hear it. (Lawson 1998, p.30)

It is not uncommon among autistic people to experience so-called daydreams. Whether this phenomenon is sixth sense, clairvoyance, precognition or any other form of so-called ESP and whether we can explain it or not, it does exist. Personal accounts of autistic individuals contain a number of these experiences, for example:

At school strange things were happening. I would have daydreams in which I was watching children I knew. I would see them doing the trivialest of things: peeling potatoes over the sink, getting themselves a peanut butter sandwich before going to bed. Such daydreams were like films in which I'd see a sequence of everyday events, which really didn't relate in any way to myself. I began to test the truth of these daydreams; approaching the friends I'd seen in them and asking them to give me a step-by-step detailed picture of what they were doing at the time I had the daydream. Amazingly, to the finest detail, I had been right. This was nothing I had controlled, it simply came into my head, but it frightened me. (Williams 1999b, pp.65–66).

Here is an example of déjà vu:

As a small boy, I often experienced the sensation of déjà vu. It manifested in a sudden realization that what was occurring in the moment had already been experienced exactly the same way once before. I also used to see things move out of the corner of my eye, or have prophetic dreams like the one in which I picked countless pennies up off our front lawn and, the next day in reality, did just that – wondering how on earth the coins got there to begin with. (Stillman 2006, p.4)

[In New York, Donna] was met by...[her] American editor. We had arrived at a huge hotel opposite Central Park... As I entered the room on the fifteenth floor, it was just sunset... I had brought my paintings along with me... Among them was a copy of the painting I had given my solicitor. It was a day scene with a hazy blue and purple sky, with the lights of the buildings playing in the reflection of the water stretching out before them. I raced to the window with my picture. My heart was thumping. Fifteen stories up, I found I had painted the scene outside of my window, building for building, steeple for steeple, in the same order, complete with the cranes now towering over them in the process of construction work. There was one thing wrong. I had painted the picture four months before coming to New York and I had never been there before. (Williams 1999c, p.159)

Whether we can explain these phenomena or not (or whether we just dismiss them as coincidences), they do exist and are very real for those who live with them. Perhaps we could follow the example of those anthropologists (see Goulet and Miller 2007; Goulet and Young 1994) who take the extraordinary experiences of the cultures they study seriously and appreciate that there are alternative ways of perceiving the world. They go beyond a traditional (and safe) cultural and academic approach and believe in the importance of reporting and reflecting on the 'paradoxical, extraordinary, shocking or baffling' experiences they encounter during fieldwork (Gardner 2007, p.17). Through long-term ethnographical fieldwork, researchers get to experience the world from the native's perspective. Since 'these accounts are based on real experiences of the researchers, and echo the experiences of their social actors (or members) in the field', they should be taken seriously, and should not be 'conceptualized (and indeed criticized) as "going native" types of story' (Coffey 1999, p.33). Whatever we choose to make of these experiences, we need to recognize that they are part of the everyday life of many people with ASDs, and that if those people are to be able to participate fully in wider society we have to accept the validity of those experiences for them.

Notes

1. This is just another reminder that some people are better at certain abilities than others.

2. They collected the sweat of novice sky-divers and samples of 'fear-free' sweat and asked volunteers to sniff the samples while having brain scans: 'fear sweat' corresponded to more activity in the brain centres.

3. Another amazing ability is sensing serious illness in their owners, or their approaching death.

4. Sheldrake calls premonition, common in animals and 'Stone Age' people (some tribes), a 'precognitive flash' – a flash of insight into the future. Modern man, Sheldrake claims, has lost much of this ability. Stillman (2006) calls it a Gift of Prophecy.

5. These experiences have been reported throughout history and across different cultures (e.g. Rhine 1969; Radin 1998). A meta-analysis of all 'forced-choice' precognition experiments (309 studies) conducted between 1935 and 1987 was published in 1989 (Honorton and Ferrari 1989). Radin hypothesizes that precognition and time-reversed effects may underlie some experiences of déjà vu, intuitive hunches, and synchronicities.

6. The research of the system of sensing might be useful.

AFTERWORD

I would like to ask for a request for more research into the different ways to perceive. Things are being broadcast to us all the time, even our own consciousnesses. I don't think there is another thing in our near solar system which can perceive in so many ways as humans can. Olga's book opens the door to a new way of understanding differences in perception. When a glass is smashed, it has experienced an action. It can only perceive this action once. But we can perceive action many times over. As substances expand and contract it is also a perception of heat being broadcast. Human perceptions are no different. There are many ways to perceive and many ways to communicate based on the different ways of perception. This could be a new area of study.

It came as quite a shock when I was diagnosed with high-functioning autism or Asperger syndrome as an adult. Books and seminars for the NT (neurotypical) audience were available to me. Very soon my inflexible behaviour, which had been a source of great distress to both me and others, started to make sense. But the general expert approach was all very mechanistic. The spectrum idea seemed to excuse apparent contradictions; *this* was a symptom I had, *that* was not. But as I was able to get along well with other autistic people, to a certain extent I was left thinking that perhaps there were things that NTs would simply never understand about me, and likewise that I would never understand about them. I remember my psychiatrist being quite baffled as I was trying to explain to him how if he closed his eyes and clicked his fingers he could see the shape of the room through sound. It was the first time in my life I realized that perceptions I had assumed other people could do all my life were perhaps unique to me. Perhaps things which were never spoken about were not spoken about because they were so basic, or maybe because the experiences were not shared.

'If you want to leave your body, just start falling asleep and then stop before you start to dream. You can get up and start walking around,' I explained to the Dalai Lama's entourage in Nottingham. Some Buddhist novices were in enthusiastic agreement while the greatest Lamas were baffled at explanations perceived as the blather of yet another deranged individual seeking an audience with his holiness. How many times in internet discussions have I made a blunt simple statement about spirituality as fact, which has met with immediate offence at the idea that mysteries pondered for centuries could have such simple explanations? But perhaps they do. Perhaps people are so desperate to retrieve that childlike sense of mystery that they miss the real magic all around us all the time. Olga's book here is, I think, the first probe into this magical 'autistic' perception of what NTs call 'mundane' reality. And I think it will help some people to discover the 'autistic' perception that they themselves can open up to if they are willing to give up on magic and open their eyes to what is already surrounding them. I was always interested in illusion as a child because, although I could see how it was done, I was amazed at the effect these tricks had on audiences. The huge emotional reactions I saw in them were great, and I learned magic in order to see the same reactions.

Now several years on I see that courses are now available to develop bat sonar. I am glad to see that not only do people now accept that different sensory realities exist, but they are open to try to learn how these might be acquired from the person next door rather than a trip across the Himalayas. Olga's book is not so much a how-to but is a much needed introduction to the science behind these alternate states of perception. For the first time it seems here is a document which challenges the conventions and says that not all humans experience reality the same way, and moreover it goes into providing a scientific basis for what critics would surely call a claim. I have been told that I can not experience reality the way NTs can; here is a well-formulated response I am glad for people to use on my behalf. You can't experience things the way I do. But, just as I want to cross that bridge and want to learn how you experience the world, if you can just be patient with me long enough to understand where I am having trouble and find the right way to explain things to me, I think you too can learn how to experience the world in the way I do, if I can also find the right way to communicate with you. I hope this book might be a springboard to provide the intellectual background for people who are interested in launching into a journey of experimentation of the different ways to perceive reality that will characterize this century.

Thank you Olga!

Kazik Hubert
An Aspie PhD student of Noachite Religion under the supervision of Dan Cohn-Sherbok at the University of Wales, Lampeter, UK

REFERENCES

Adams, V. (2002) 'Randomised controlled crime: Postcolonial sciences in alternative medicine research.' *Social Studies of Science 32*, (5–6), 659–690.

Adler, L.E., Waldo, M.C. and Freedman, R. (1985) 'Neurophysiologic studies of sensory gating in schizophrenia: Comparison of auditory and visual responses.' *Biological Psychiatry 20*, 1284–1296.

Alford, Dan Moonhawk (1994) 'Pinker's book and linguist bashing.' Available from http://linguistlist.org/issues/5/5-768.html#1, accessed on 22 March 2010.

Alford, Dan Moonhawk (2002) 'The great Whorf hypothesis hoax: Sin, suffering and redemption in academe.' Chapter 7 in *The Secret Life of Language*, 17 October 2010 draft. Available from www.enformy.com/dma-Chap7.htm, accessed on 22 March 2010.

Alibali, M.W., Heath, D.C. and Myers, H.J. (2001) 'Effects of visibility between speaker and listener on gesture production: Some gestures are meant to be seen.' *Neuropsychologia 44*, 161–170.

Allen, G. and Courchesne, E. (2003) 'Differential effects of developmental cerebellar abnormality on cognitive and motor functions in cerebellum: An fMRI study of autism.' *American Journal of Psychiatry 160*, 262–273.

Allen, G., Muller, R.A. and Courchesne, E. (2004) 'Cerebellar function in autism: Functional magnetic resonance image activation during a simple motor task.' *Biological Psychiatry 56*, 269–278.

Alvarez, A. (1972) *The Savage God: A Study of Suicide.* New York: Random House.

Armstrong-Buck, S. (1989) 'Nonhuman experience: A Whiteheadian analysis.' *Process Studies 18*, 1, 1–18.

Ashwin, E., Ashwin, C., Rhydderch, D., Howells, J. and Baron-Cohen, S. (2009) 'Eagle-eyed acuity: Experimental investigation of enhanced perception in autism.' *Biological Psychiatry 65*, 1, 17–21.

Asperger, H. (1944) 'Die "Autistischen Psychopathen" im Kindesalter.' *Archiv fur Psychiatrie und Nervenkrankheiten 117*, 76–136.

Atkinson, J.M. (1992) 'Shamanism today.' *Annual Review of Anthropology 21*, 307–330.

Banissy, M.J. and Ward, J. (2007) 'Mirror Touch synesthesia is linked with empathy.' *Nature Neuroscience 10*, 815–816.

Barbour, A. (1976) *Louder than Words: Non-Verbal Communication*. Columbus, OH: Charles E. Merill Publishing Company.

Barsalou, L.W. (1999) 'Perceptual symbol systems.' *Behavioral and Brain Sciences 22*, 577–609.

Baruth, J.M., Casanova, M.F., Sears, L. and Sokhadze, E. (In press) 'Early visual processing abnormalities in autism spectrum disorders.' *Autism Research and Treatment.*

Bauman, M.L. and Kemper, T.L. (1994) *The Neurobiology of Autism*. Baltimore, MD: The Hopkins University Press.

Bauman, M.L. and Kemper, T.L. (2005) 'Neuroanatomic observations of the brain in autism: A review and future directions.' *International Journal of Developmental Neuroscience 23*, 2–3, 183–187.

Becklen, R. and Cervone, D. (1983) 'Selective looking and the noticing of unexpected events.' *Memory and Cognition 11*, 601–608.

Belenky, M.F., Clinchy, B.M., Goldberg, N.R. and Tarule, J.M. (1986) *Women's Ways of Knowing: The Development of Self, Voice and Mind*. New York: Basic Books.

Benarik, R.G., Lewis-Williams, J.D. and Dowson, T.A. (1990) 'On neuropsychology and shamanism in rock art.' *Current Anthropology 31*, 1, 77–84.

Bergman, P. and Escalona, S.K. (1949) 'Unusual sensitivities in very young children.' *Psychoanalytical Study of the Child 3/4*, 333–352.

Bergson, H. (1911/1944) *Creative Evolution*. New York: The Modern Library.

Bergson, H. (1911) 'Life and consciousness.' *The Hibbert Journal X*, October 1911, 24–44.

Bergson, H. (1912/1999) *An Introduction to Metaphysics*. Indianapolis, IN/Cambridge: Hackett Publishing Company.

Berlin, B. and Kay, P. (1969) *Basic Color Terms: Their Universality and Evolution*. Berkeley, CA: University of California Press.

Biklen, D. (1990) 'Communication unbound: Autism and praxis.' *Harvard Educational Review 60*, 291–314.

Biklen, D. (1992) 'Facilitated Communication: Biklen responds.' *American Journal of Speech and Language Pathology 2*, 21–22.

Bion, W.R. (1963) *Elements of Psycho-Analysis*. London: Heinemann.

Bird, G., Leighton, J., Press, C. and Heyes, C.M. (2007) 'Intact automatic imitation of human and robot actions in autism spectrum disorders.' *Proceedings and Biological Sciences 274*, 3027–3031.

Blackburn, J. (1999) *My Inside View of Autism*. www.planet.com/urers/blackjar/aisub (site no longer active), accessed on 5 December 2002.

Blackman, L. (2001) *Lucy's Story: Autism and Other Adventures*. London: Jessica Kingsley Publishers.

Blakemore, S.J., Bristow, D., Bird, G., Frith, C. and Ward, J. (2005) 'Somatosensory observations during the observation of touch and a case of vision-touch synaesthesia.' *Brain 128*, 1571–1583.

Blakemore, S.J., Tavassoli, T., Thomas, R.M., Catmur, C., Frith, U. and Haggard, P. (2006) 'Tactile sensitivity in Asperger syndrome.' *Brain and Cognition 61*, 5–13.

Block, J.R. and Yuker, H.E. (1989) *Can You Believe Your Eyes?* London: Routledge.

Bogdashina, O. (2003) *Sensory Perceptual Issues in Autism and Asperger Syndrome: Different Sensory Experiences – Different Perceptual Worlds*. London: Jessica Kingsley Publishers.

Bogdashina, O. (2004) *Communication Issues in Autism and Asperger Syndrome: Do We Speak the Same Language?* London: Jessica Kingsley Publishers.

Bogdashina, O. (2005) *Theory of Mind and the Triad of Perspectives on Autism and Asperger Syndrome: A View from the Bridge*. London: Jessica Kingsley Publishers.

Bogdashina, O. (2006) 'Autistic accounts of sensory-perceptual experiences: Should we listen?' *Good Autism Practice 7*, 3–12.

Bogoras, W. (1907) *The Chukchee. Part II. The Jessup North Pacific Expedition*, Vol. 7. New York: G.E. Techert.

Bornstein, M.H. (1987) 'Perceptual Categories in Vision and Audition.' In S. Harnad (ed.) *Categorical Perception: The Groundwork of Cognition*. New York: Cambridge University Press.

Boroditsky, L. (2009) 'How does our language shape the way we think?' In M. Brockman (ed.) *What's Next? Dispatches on the Future of Science*, 116–129. New York: Vintage Books.

Bourguignon, E. (1976) *Possession*. San Francisco, CA: Chandler and Sharp.

Boutros, N., Kozuukov, O., Jansen, B., Feingold, A. and Bell, M. (2004) 'Sensory gating deficits during the mid-latency phase of information processing in medicated schizophrenia patents.' *Psychiatry Research 126*, 203–215.

Boyer, L.B. (1962) 'Remarks on the personality of shamans, with special reference to the Apache of the Mescalero Indian Reservation.' *Psychoanalytic Study of Society 2*, 233–254.

Boyer, L.B. (1964) 'Further remarks concerning shamans and shamanism' *Isreal Annals of Psychiatry and Related disciples 2*, 3, 235–257.

Boyer, L.B. (1969) 'Shamans: to set the record straight.' *American Anthropology 71*, 307–309.

Browman, D.L. and Schwartz, R.A. (1979) *Spirits, Shamans, and Stars: Perspectives from South America*. The Hague: Mouton.

Brown, D. (2006) *Tricks of the Mind*. London: Channel 4 Books.

Brown, R.W. (1958) *Words and Things*. Glencoe, IL: Free Press.

Brown, R. and Lennenberg, E.H. (1954) 'A study in language and cognition.' *Journal of Abnormal and Social Psychology 49*, 454–462.

Brown, R.E. and Milner, P.M. (2003) 'The legacy of Donald O. Hebb: More than the Hebb Synapse.' *Nature Reviews Neuroscience 4*, 1013–1019.

Bucci, W. (1997) 'Symptoms and symbols: A multiple code theory of somatization.' *Psychoanalytic Inquiry 2*, 151–172.

Bufalari, I., Aprile, T., Avenanti, A., Di Russo, F. and Aglioty, S.M. (2007) 'Empathy for pain and touch in the human cerebral cortex.' *Cerebral Cortex 17*, 2553–2561.

Carroll, J.B. (1956) 'Introduction' to B.L. Whorf. *Language, Thought and Reality*. Cambridge, MA: MIT Press.

Casanova, M.F. (2004) 'White matter volume increase and minicolumns in autism.' *Annals of Neurology 56*, 3, 453.

Casanova, M.F. (2006) 'Brains of the autistic individuals.' *International AWARE On-Line Conference Papers*. Available at www.autism2006.org, access via registration only.

Casanova, M.F. (2009) Personal communication (email), 6 November 2009.

Casanova, M.F., Buxhoeveden, D.P. and Brown, C. (2002a) 'Clinical and macroscopic correlates of minicolumnar pathology in autism.' *Journal of Child Neurology 17*, 692–695.

Casanova, M.F., Buxhoeveden, D.P. and Gomez, J. (2003) 'Disruption in the inhibitory architecture of the cell minicolumn: Implication for autism.' *Neuroscientist 9*, 496–507.

Casanova, M.F., Buxhoeveden, D.P., Switala, A.E. and Roy, E. (2002b) 'Minicolumnar pathology in autism.' *Neurology 58*, 428–432.

Casanova, M.F. and Switala. A.E. (2005) 'Minicolumnar morphometry: computerized image analysis.' In M.F. Casanova (ed.) *Neocortical Modularity and the Cell Minicolumn*, 161–179. New York: Nova Biomedical Books.

Cascio, C. McGlone, F., Folger, S., Tannan, V., Baranek, G., Pelphrey, K.A. and Essick, G. (2008) 'Tactile perception in adults with autism: Multidimensional psychophysical study.' *Journal of Autism and Developmental Disorders 38*, 127–137.

Cass, H. (1996) 'Visual impairments and autism – What we know about causation and early identification.' Autism and Visual Impairment Conference, *Sensory Series 5*, 2–24.

Cassirer, E. (1946) *Language and Myth*. New York: Harper Brothers.

Castaneda, C. (1971) *A Separate Reality: Further Conversations with Don Juan*. New York: Simon and Schuster.

Castaneda, C. (1972) *Journey to Ixtlan: The Lessons of Don Juan*. New York: Simon and Schuster.

Castaneda, C. (1974) *Tales of Power*. New York: Simon and Schuster.

Castaneda, C. (1998) *The Wheel of Time*. New York: Washington Square Press.

Castiello, U., Paulignan, Y. and Jeannerod, M. (1991) 'Temporal dissociation of motor responses and subjective awareness.' *Brain 114*, 2639–2655.

Charles, M. (1999) 'Patterns: Unconscious shaping of self and experience.' *J. M. Klein and Objects Relations 17*, 367–388.

Charles, M. (2001) 'A "confusion of tongues": Difficulties in conceptualizing development in psychoanalytic theories.' *Human Nature Review*, 28 March, www. human-nature.com/ksej/charles.htm (site no longer active), accessed on 8 October 2002.

Chase, S. (1956) 'Foreword.' In B.L. Whorf. *Language, Thought and Reality*. Cambridge, MA: MIT Press.

Chomsky, N. (1957) *Syntactic Structures*. The Hague: Mouton Publishers.

Clark, A. (2002) 'Is Seeing All It Seems?' In A. Noe (ed.) *Is the Visual World a Grand Illusion?* Exeter: Imprint Academic.

Clarke, A.C. (2000) *Profiles of the Future: An Inquiry into the Limits of the Possible* (Millennium Edition). London: Indigo.

Coates, P. (2003) 'Review of *Is the Visual World a Grand Illusion?' Human Nature Review 3*, 176–182.

Coffey, A. (1999) *The Ethnographic Self, Fieldwork and Representation of Identity*. London: Sage.

Cohen, L.B. (1991) 'Infant Attention: An Information Processing Approach.' In M.J. Zelazo (ed.) *Newborn Attention: Biological Constraints and the Influence of Experience.* 1–21. Norwood, NJ: Ablex.

Corbett, J. (2000) *Jungle Law*, 2nd edition. New Delhi: Oxford University Press.

Courchesne, E. (2002) 'Abnormal early brain development in autism.' *Molecular Psychiatry 7*, Suppl. 2, S21–S23.

Courchesne, E. (2004) 'Brain development in autism: Early overgrowth followed by premature arrest of growth.' *Mental Retardation and Developmental Disabilities Research Reviews 10*, 106–111.

Courchesne, E. and Pierce, K. (2005) 'Why the frontal cortex in autism might be talking only to itself: Local over-connectivity but long-distance disconnection.' *Current Opinion in Neurobiology 15*, 225–230.

Courtenay-Smith, N. (2008) 'Imagine spending 48 hours locked in a pitch black bunker with no human contact. This man did it – and he almost lost his mind.' *Daily Mail*, 22 January 2008; BBC2 documentary.

Cowey, A. and Stoerig, P. (1991) 'The neurology of blindsight.' *Trends in Neuroscience 14*, 140–145.

Creak, M. (1961) 'Schizophrenia syndrome in childhood: Progress report of a working party.' *Cerebral Palsy Bulletin 3*, 501–504.

Crossley, R. (1992) 'Getting the words out: Case studies in facilitated communication training.' *Topics in Language Disorders 12*, 46–59.

Crossley, R. (1993) 'Flying high on paper wings.' *Journal of International Exchange of Experts and Information of Rehabilitation 4*, April, 21–110.

Czaplika, M.A. (1914) *Aboriginal Siberia.* Oxford: Oxford University Press.

Damasio, A.R. (1989) 'Time-locked multiregional retroactivation: A systems-level proposal for the neural substrates of recall and recognition.' *Cognition 33*, 1–2, 25–62.

Damasio, A.R. and Damasio, H. (1994) 'Cortical Systems for Retrieval of Concrete Knowledge: The Convergence Zone Framework.' In C. Loch and J.L. Davis (eds) *Large-Scale Neuronal Theories of the Brain.* Cambridge, MA: MIT Press.

Dapretto, M., Davies, M.S., Pfeifer, J.H., Scott, A.A., Sigman, M., Bookheimer, S.Y. and Iacoboni, M. (2006) 'Understanding emotions in others: Mirror neuron dysfunction in children with autism spectrum disorders.' *Nature Neuroscience 9*, 28–30.

Daria, T.O. (2008) *Dasha's Journal: A Cat Reflects on Life, Catness and Autism.* London: Jessica Kingsley Publishers.

Darwin, C. (1872) *The Expression of the Emotions in Man and Animals.* London: Murray.

Davis, P.C.W. (1984) *Superforce.* London: Heinemann.

Davis, T., Hoffman, D. and Rodriguez, A. (2002) 'Visual Worlds: Construction and Reconstruction.' In A. Noe (ed.) *Is the Visual World a Grand Illusion?* Exeter: Imprint Academic.

Dean, D. and Nash, C.B. (1963) 'Plethysmograph Results under Strict Conditions.' *Sixth Annual Convention of the Parapsychological Association*, New York.

Deeley, Q. (2009) 'Pathophysiology of autism: Evidence from brain imaging.' *British Journal of Hospital Medicine 70*, 3, 138–142.

Delacato, C. (1974) *The Ultimate Stranger: The Autistic Child.* Noveto, CA: Academic Therapy Publications.

DeMille, R. (1976) *Castaneda's Journey.* Santa Barbara: Capra Press.

Dennett, D.C. (1992) 'Temporal Anomalies of Consciousness.' In Y. Christen and P.S. Churchland (eds) *Neurophilosophy and Alzheimer's Disease.* Berlin: Springer-Verlag.

Dennett, D.C. (1994) 'The Role of Language in Intelligence.' In J. Khalfa (ed.) *What Is Intelligence?* Cambridge: Cambridge University Press.

Dennett, D.C. and Kinsbourne, M. (1992) 'Time and the observer: The where and when of consciousness in the brain.' *Behavioral and Brain Sciences 15,* 183–247.

De Quincey, T. (1821/1967) *Confessions of an English Opium-Eater.* London: Dent.

d'Espagnat, B. (1973) 'Conceptual Foundations of Quantum Mechanics.' In J. Mehra (ed.) *The Physicist's Conception of Nature.* Boston, MA: Kluwer.

Devereux, G. (1961) 'Shamans as neurotics.' *American Anthropology 63,* 1088–1090.

Dobkin di Rios, M. and Winkelman, M. (1989) 'Shamanism and altered states of consciousness.' *Journal of Psychoactive Drugs 21,* 1.

Doman, R.J. (1984) 'Sensory deprivation.' *National Association for the Child Development 4,* 3, 4–5.

Donald, M. (1991) *Origins of the Modern Mind: Three Stages in the Evolution of Culture and Cognition.* Cambridge, MA: Harvard University Press.

Douglas, V.I. and Peters, K.G. (1979) 'Towards a Clearer Definition of Attention Deficit of Hyperactive Children.' In G.A. Hale and M. Lewis (eds) *Attention and Cognitive Development.* New York: Plenum Press.

Dunbar, R. (1996) *Grooming Gossip and the Evolution of Language.* Cambridge, MA: Harvard University Press.

Eagleman, D.M. and Sejnowski, T. (2000) 'Motion integration and postdiction in visual awareness.' *Science 287,* 2036–2038.

Eddington, A. (1958) *Philosophy of Physical Science.* East Lansing, MI: University of Michigan Press.

Ekman, P. and Friesen, W. (1969) 'Nonverbal leakage and cues to deception.' *Psychiatry 32,* 88–106.

Ekman, P. and Friesen, W. (1972) 'Hand movements.' *Journal of Communication 22,* 353–374.

Eveloff, H.H. (1960) 'The autistic child.' *Archives of General Psychiatry 3,* 66–81.

Farah, M.J. (1989) 'The neural basis of mental imagery.' *Trends in Neuroscience 12,* 395–399.

Farah, M.J. and Feinberg, T.E. (1997) 'Perception and Awareness.' In T.E. Feinberg and M.J. Farah (eds) *Behavioral Neurology and Neuropsychology.* New York: McGraw-Hill.

Fay, W. and Schuler, A. (1980) *Emerging Language in Children with Autism.* Baltimore, MD: University Park Press.

Feigenberg, I.M. (1986) *To See – to Predict – to Act.* Moscow: Znanie. (In Russian.)

Fernandez-Duque, D. and Thornton, I.M. (2000) 'Change detection without awareness: Do explicit reports underestimate the representation of change in the visual system?' *Visual Cognition 7,* 324–344.

Feuer, L. (1953) 'Sociological aspects of the relation between language and philosophy.' *Philosophy of Science 20,* 85–100.

Fikes, J.C. (1993) *Carlos Castaneda: Academic Opportunism and Psychedelic Sixties*. Victoria: Millennia Press.

Flavell, J.H., Everett, B.A., Croft, K. and Flavell, E.R. (1981) 'Young children's knowledge about visual perception: Further evidence for the Level 1–Level 2 distinction.' *Developmental Psychology 17*, 99–103.

Forrest, D. (ed.) (1996) *A Glimpse of Hell*. London: Amnesty International.

Freedman, R., Adler, L., Gerhardt, G., Waldo, M., Baker, N., Rose, G., *et al.* (1987) 'Neurobiological studies of sensory gating in schizophrenia.' *Schizophrenia Bulletin 13*, 669–678.

Freedman, R., Olincy, A., Ross, R.G., Waldo, M.C., Stevens, K.E., Adler, L.E., *et al.* (2003) 'The genetics of sensory gating deficits in schizophrenia.' *Current Psychiatry 5*, 155–161.

Frith, U. (2003) *Autism: Explaining the Enigma*, 2nd edition. Oxford: Blackwell Publishing.

Furst, P.T. (1972) *Flesh of the Gods: The Ritual Use of Hallucinogens*. New York: Praeger.

Gainotti, G., Silveri, M.C., Daniele, A. and Giustolisi, L. (1995) 'Neuroanatomical correlates of category-specific semantic disorders: A critical survey.' *Memory 3*, 247–264.

Gardner, P.M. (2007) 'On Puzzling Wavelengths.' In J.-G. Goulet and B.G. Miller (2007) (eds) *Extraordinary Anthropology: Transformations in the Field*. Lincoln and London: University of Nebraska Press.

Gazzaniga, M.S. (1988) 'Brain modularity: Towards a Philosophy of Conscious Experience.' In A.J. Marcel and E. Bisiach (eds) *Consciousness in Contemporary Science*. Oxford: Clarendon Press.

Gense, M.H. and Gense, D.J. (1994) 'Identifying autism in children with blindness and visual impairment.' *Review 26*, 56–62.

Gibson, E.J. (1969) *Principles of Perceptual Learning and Perceptual Development*. New York: Appleton Century Croft.

Goldstein, G., Beers, S.R., Siegel, D.J. and Minshew, N.J. (2001) 'A comparison of WAIS-R profiles in adults with high-functioning autism or differing subtypes of learning disability.' *Applied Neuropsychology 8*, 148–154.

Goodale, M.A. (1993) 'Visual routes to knowledge and action.' *Biomedical Research, 14*, 113–123.

Goodman, F.D. (1990) *Where the Spirits Ride the Wind: Trance Journey and Other Ecstatic Experiences*. Bloomington, IN: Indiana University Press.

Goulet, J.-G. and Miller, B.G. (2007) (eds) *Extraordinary Anthropology: Transformations in the Field*. Lincoln and London: University of Nebraska Press.

Goulet, J.G. and Young, D.E. (1994) (eds) *Being Changed by Cross-Cultural Encounters: The Anthropology of Extraordinary Experience*. Peterborough, ON: Broadview Press.

Grandin, T. (1996a) *Thinking in Pictures and Other Reports from My Life with Autism*. New York: Vintage Books.

Grandin, T. (1996b) 'My experiences with visual thinking, sensory problems and communication difficulties.' Centre for the Study of Autism. Accessed at www.autism.org/temple/visual.html (site no longer active), on 8 October 2002.

Grandin, T. (1998) 'Consciousness in animals and people with autism.' Available from www.grandin.com, accessed on 22 March 2010.

Grandin, T. (2000) 'My mind is a web browser: How people with autism think.' *Cerebrum 2*, 1, 14–22.

Grandin, T. (2008) *The Way I See It: A Personal Look at Autism and Asperger's.* Arlington, TX: Future Horizons.

Grandin, T. and Johnson, C. (2005) *Animals in Translation: Using the Mysteries of Autism to Decode Animal Behavior.* London: Bloomsbury.

Gregory, R. (1997) 'Editorial: Doors of perception.' *Perception 26*, 1.

Gribbin, J. (1991) *In Search of Schrodinger's Cat: Quantum Physics and Reality.* London: Black Swan.

Gunn, J.A. (1920) *Bergson and His Philosophy.* Available from www.ibiblio.org/ HTMLTexts/John_Alexander_Gunn/Bergson_And_His_Philosophy, accessed on 22 March 2010.

Gurney, C. (2001) *The Language of Animals: 7 Steps to Communicating with Animals.* New York: The Bantam Dell Publishing Group.

Hadjikhani, N., Joseph, R.M., Snyder, J. and Flusberg, H. (2007) 'Abnormal activation of the social brain during face perception in autism.' *Human Brain Mapping 28*, 441–449.

Hamilton, A.F., Brindley, R.M. and Frith, U. (2007) 'Imitation and action understanding in autistic spectrum disorders: How valid is the hypothesis of a deficit in the mirror neuron system?' *Neuropsychologia 45*, 1859–1868.

Handelman, D. (1967) 'The development of a Washo shaman.' *Ethnology 6*, 4, 444–464.

Happe, F. (1999) 'Autism: cognitive deficit or cognitive style.' *Trends in Cognitive Science 3*, 216–222.

Harnad, S. (1987) 'The Induction and Representation of Categories.' In S. Harnad (ed.) *Categorical Perception: The Groundwork of Cognition.* New York: Cambridge University Press.

Harnad, S. (1996) 'The Origin of Words: A Psychophysical Hypothesis.' In B. Velichkovsky and D. Rumbaugh (eds) *Communicating Meaning: Evolution and Development of Language.* NJ: Erlbaum.

Harner, M.J. (1973) *Hallucinogens and Shamanism.* Oxford: Oxford University Press.

Hartman, B.O. and Secrist, G.E. (1991) 'Situational awareness is more than exceptional vision.' *Aviation, Space, and Environmental Medicine 62*, 11, 1084–1089.

Haskew, P. and Donnellan, A. (1993) *Emotional Maturity and Well-Being: Psychological Lessons of Facilitated Communication.* Madison, WI: DRI Press.

Hatfield, E., Cacioppo, J. and Rapson, R. (1994) *Emotional Contagion.* Cambridge: Cambridge University Press.

Hawthorne, D. (2002) 'My common sense approach to autism.' *Autism Today*, Available from www.autismtoday.com/articles/commonsense.htm, accessed on 22 March 2010.

Hay, D.F. (1994) 'Prosocial development.' *Journal of Child Psychology and Psychiatry and Allied Disciplines 35*, 29–71.

Heisenberg, W. (1927) 'Uber den anschaulichen Inhalt der quantentheoretischen Kinematik und Mechanik.' *Zeitschrift fur Physik 43*, 172–198. (Trans. John Gribbin.)

Hermelin, B. (2001) *Bright Splinters of the Mind: A Personal Story of Research with Autistic Savants.* London: Jessica Kingsley Publishers.

Hermelin, B. and O'Connor, N. (1990) 'Art and accuracy: The drawing ability of idiot-savants.' *Journal of Child Psychology and Psychiatry 31*, 217–228.

Hill, A.A. (1958) *Introduction to Linguistic Structures.* New York: Harcourt.

Hjelmslev, L. (1961) *Prolegomena to a Theory of Language.* Madison, WI: University of Wisconsin Press. (Trans. F.J. Whitfield.)

Hoijer, H. (1953) 'The Relation of Language to Culture.' In A.L. Kroeber (ed.) *Anthropology Today,* 554–573. Chicago, IL: University of Chicago Press.

Honorton, C. and Ferrari, D.C. (1989) 'Future telling: A meta-analysis of forced-choice precognition experiments, 1935–1987.' *Journal of Parapsychology 53*, 281–308.

Horowitz, A. (2007) 'Why endless politically correct legislation has been the death of the villain.' *Daily Mail,* 5 June 2007.

Humphrey, N. (1992) *A History of the Mind: Evolution and the Birth of Consciousness.* London: Chatto and Windus.

Humphrey, N. (1998) 'Cave art, autism, and the evolution of the human mind.' *Cambridge Archaeological Journal 8*, 2, 165–191.

Humphrey, N. (2002) 'Thinking about feeling.' In G. Richard (ed.) *Oxford Companion to the Mind.* New York: Oxford University Press.

Huxley, A. (1954/2004) 'The Doors of Perception.' London: Vintage.

Huxley, A. (1956/2004) 'Heaven and Hell.' London: Vintage.

Innes-Smith, M. (1987) 'Pre-oedipal identification and the cathexis of autistic object in the aetiology of adult psychopathology.' *International Journal of Psycho-Analysis 68*, 405–413.

Inoue, S. and Matsuzawa, T. (2007) 'Working memory of numerals in chimpanzees.' *Current Biology 17*, 23, R1004–R1005.

Isaacson, R. (2009) *The Horse Boy: A Father's Miraculous Journey to Heal His Son.* London: Viking.

Jackson, P.L., Brunet, E., Meltzoff, A.N. and Decety, J. (2006) 'Empathy examined through the neural mechanisms involved in imaging how I feel versus how you feel pain.' *Neuropsychologia 44*, 752–761.

Joan and Rich (1999) 'What is autism?' Accessed at www.ani.autistics.org/joan_rich. html (site no longer active), on 18 January 2000.

Johansson, M., Rastam, M., Billstedt, E., Danielsson, S., Stromland, K. and Miller, M. (2006) 'Autism spectrum disorders and underlying brain pathology in CHARGE association.' *Developmental Medicine and Child Neurology 48*, 40–50.

Johnson-Laird, P.N. (1983) *Mental Models: Towards a Cognitive Science of Language, Inference and Consciousness.* Cambridge, MA: Harvard University Press.

Johnson-Laird, P.N. (1989) 'Analogy and the exercise of creativity.' In S. Vosniadou and A. Ortony (eds) *Similarity and Analogical Reasoning.* Cambridge: Cambridge University Press.

Jolliffe, T. and Baron-Cohen, S. (1997) 'Are people with autism and Asperger syndrome faster than normal on the embedded figures test?' *Child Psychology and Psychiatry 38*, 527–534.

Jones, S.S. and Smith, L.B. (1993) 'The place of perception in children's concepts.' *Cognitive Development 8*, 113–139.

Joralemon, D. (1984) 'The role of hallucinogenic drugs and sensory stimuli in Peruvian ritual healing.' *Culture, Medicine and Psychology 8*, 399–430.

Jung, C.G. (1923) *Psychological Types*. New York: Harcourt Brace and World.

Jung, C.G. (1958) *The Undiscovered Self*. London: Routledge.

Just, M.A., Cherkassky, V.L., Keller, T.A. and Minshew, N.J. (2004) 'Cortical activation, synchronization during sentence comprehension in high-functioning autism: Evidence of underconnectivity.' *Brain 127*, 1811–1821.

Kaffman, A. and Meaney, M.J. (2007) 'Neurodevelopmental sequelae of postnatal maternal care in rodents: Clinical and research implications of molecular insights.' *Journal of Child Psychology and Psychiatry 48*, 224–244.

Kahneman, D., Treisman, A. and Gibbs, B. (1992) 'The reviewing of object files: Object-specific integration of information.' *Cognitive Psychology 24*, 175–219.

Kana, R.K., Keller, T.A., Cherkassky, V.L., Minshew, N.J. and Just, M.A. (2006) 'Sentence comprehension in autism: Thinking in pictures with decreased functional connectivity.' *Brain 129*, 2484–2493.

Kanner, L. (1943) 'Autistic disturbances of affective contact.' *Nervous Child 2*, 217–250.

Kaplan, L. (2003) 'Inuit snow terms: How many and what does it mean?' In: *Building Capacity in Arctic Societies: Dynamics and shifting perspectives. Proceedings from the 2nd IPSSAS Seminar*. Iqaluit, Nunavut, Canada: 26 May–6 June, 2003. Available from http://www.uaf.edu/anlc/snow.html, accessed on 22 March 2010.

Kaptchuk, T.J. (1998) 'Powerful placebo: The dark side of the randomised controlled trial.' *The Lancet 351*, 9117, 1722–1725.

Khalfa, S., Bruneau, N., Roge, B., Georgieff, N., Vevillet, E., Adrien, J.L. *et al.* (2004) 'Increased perception of loudness in autism.' *Hearing Research 198*, 87–92.

Kimball, M. (2005) *Interpretations of the Mind: An Exploration of Consciousness and Autism*. Availble from www.autism-society.org/site/DocServer/Interpretations_of_the_Mind.pdf?doc%5C, accessed on 22 March 2010.

King, C.D. (1963) *The State of Human Consciousness*. New York: University Books.

Kluckhohn, C. (1954) 'Culture and Behavior.' In G. Lindzey (ed.) *Handbook of Social Psychology*. Cambridge, MA: Addison-Wesley Press.

Kluckhohn, C. and Leighton, D. (1946) *The Novaho*. Cambridge, MA: Harvard University Press.

Kochmeister, S. (1995) 'Excerpts from "Shattering Walls".' *Facilitated Communication Digest 5*, 3, 9–11.

Koshino, H., Carpenter, P.A., Minshew, N.J., Cherkassky, V.L., Keller, T.A. and Just, M.A. (2005) 'Functional connectivity in an fMRI working memory task in high-functioning autism.' *Neuroimage 24*, 810–821.

Krystal, H. (1988) *Integration and Self-Healing: Affect, Trauma, Alexithymia*. Hillsdale, NJ: Analytic.

Kumin, I. (1996) *Pre-Object Relatedness: Early Attachment and the Psychoanalytic Situation*. New York and London: Guilford Press.

LaFee, S. (2007) 'More than a feeling.' Available from http://legacy.signonsandiego.com/uniontrib/20070315/news_lz1c15senses.html, accessed on 27 April 2010.

Lane, H. (1976) *The Wild Boy of Aveyron: A History of the Education of Retarded, Deaf, and Hearing Children*. Cambridge, MA: Harvard University Press.

Lane, D.M. and Pearson, D.A. (1982) 'The development of selective attention.' *Merrill-Palmer Quarterly 28*, 317–337.

Lawrence, D.H. (1950) 'Acquired distinctiveness of cues: II. Selective association in a constant stimulus situation.' *Journal of Experimental Psychology 40*, 175–188.

Lawson, W. (1998) *Life Behind Glass: A Personal Account of Autism Spectrun Disorder.* Lismore: Southern Cross University Press.

Lawson, W. (2001) *Understanding and Working with the Spectrum of Autism: An Insider's View.* London: Jessica Kingsley Publishers.

Lee, T.W., Josephs, O., Dolan, R.J. and Critchley, H.D. (2006) 'Imitating expressions: Emotion-specific neural substrates in facial mimicry.' *Social Cognitive and Affective Neuroscience 1*, 122–135.

Levinson, S.C. (2003) *Space in Language and Cognition: Exploration in Cognitive Diversity.* New York: Cambridge University Press.

Levinson, S.C. and Wilkins, D.P. (eds) (2006) *Grammars of Space: Explorations in Cognitive Diversity.* New York: Cambridge University Press.

Levitt, P. (2005) 'Disruption of interneuron development.' *Epilepsia 46*, 7, 22–28.

Lewis-Williams, J.D. (1987) 'A dream of eland: An unexplored component of San shamanism and rock art.' *World Archaelogy 19*, 2, 165–177.

Lewis-Williams, J.D. and Dowson, T.A. (1988) 'The signs of all times: Entoptic phenomena in Upper Paleolithic art.' *Current Anthropology 29*, 2, 201–245.

Lex, B. (1979) 'The Neurology of Ritual Trance.' In E. d'Aquili (ed.) *The Spectrum of Ritual: A Biogenetic Structural Analysis.* New York: Columbia University Press.

Libet, B. (1985) 'Unconscious cerebral initiative and the role of conscious will in voluntary action.' *Behavioral and Brain Sciences 8*, 529–566.

Lieberman, M.D., Eisenberger, N.I., Crockett, M.J., Tom, S.M., Pfeifer, J.H. and Way, B.M. (2007) 'Putting feelings into words: Affect labeling disrupts amygdala activity in response to affective stimuli.' *Psychological Science 5*, 421–428.

Lilly, J.C. (1972) *Programming and Metaprogramming in the Human Biocomputer.* New York: Julian Press.

Loveland, K. (1991) 'Social affordances and interaction: Autism and affordances of the human environment.' *Ecological Psychology 3*, 99–119.

Lund, J., Angelucci, A. and Bressloff, P. (2003) 'Anatomical substrates for functional columns in macaque monkey primary visual cortex.' *Cerebral Cortex 13*, 15–24.

Mack, A. and Rock, I. (1998) *Inattentional Blindness.* Cambridge, MA: MIT Press.

Malotki, E. (1983) 'Hopi time: A linguistic analysis of the temporal concepts in the Hopi language.' *Trends in Linguistics, Studies and Monographs 20.* Berlin: Walter de Gruyter.

Mandler, J.M. (1992) 'How to build a baby: II. Conceptual primitives.' *Psychological Review 99*, 587–604.

Marcel, A.J. (1983) 'Conscious and unconscious perception: Experiments on visual masking and word recognition.' *Cognitive Psychology 15*, 197–237.

Markram, H., Rinaldi, T. and Markram, K. (2007) 'The intense world syndrome – an alternative hypothesis for autism.' *Frontiers in Neuroscience 1*, 77–96.

Martin, L. (1986) '"Eskimo words for snow": A case study in the genesis and decay of an anthropological example.' *American Anthropologist, New Series 18*, 2, 418–423.

Maslow, A.H. (1970) *Religions, Values, and Peak-Experiences*. New York: Penguin.

Matsuzawa, T. (2009) 'Q and A: Tetsuro Matsuzawa.' *Current Biology 19*, 8, R310–R312.

Matte-Blanco, I. (1975) *The Unconscious as Infinite Sets: An Essay in Bi-Logic*. London: Duckworth.

Matte-Blanco, I. (1988) *Thinking, Feeling, and Being: Clinical Reflections on the Fundamental Antinomy of Human Beings and World*. London and New York: Routledge.

McAlonan, G.M., Cheung, C., Cheung, V., Wong, N., Suckling, J. and Chua, S.E. (2009) 'Differential effects on white-matter systems in high-functioning autism and Asperger's syndrome.' *Psychological Medicine 39*, 11, 1885–1893.

McCraty, R. (2004) cited in 'Mindsight and precognition.' *JREF Online Newsletter 20*, February 2004. Available from www.randi.org/jr/022004demons.html, accessed on 19 November 2007.

McKean, T. (1994) *Soon Will Come the Light*. Arlington, TX: Future Horizons, Inc.

McKean, T. (1999) Articles. Available from www.geocites.com/-soonlight/SWCTL/ARTICLES, accessed on 23 October 2002.

McKenna, T. (1992) *The Archaic Revival: Speculations on Psychedelic Mushrooms, the Amazon, Virtual Reality, UFOs and More*. San Francisco, CA: Harper.

Merikle, P.M. and Joordens, S. (1997) 'Parallels between perception without attention and perception without awareness.' *Consciousness and Cognition 6*, 219–236.

Merikle, P.M. and Reingold, E.M. (1992) Measuring Unconscious Perceptual Processes. In R.F. Bernstein and T.S. Pittman (eds) *Perception Without Awareness*. New York: Guilford Press.

Miller, B.L., Boone, K., Cummings, J., Read, S.L. and Mishkin, F. (2000) 'Functional correlates of musical and visual ability in frontal temporal dementia.' *British Journal of Psychiatry 176*, 458–463.

Miller, B.L., Cummings, J., Mishkin, F., Boone, K., Prince, F., Ponton, M. and Cotman, C. (1998) 'Emergence of art talent in frontal temporal dementia.' *Neurology 51*, 978–982.

Miller, G.A. (1951) *Language and Communication*. New York: McGraw-Hill Book Co.

Milner, A.D. and Goodale, M.A. (1995) *The Visual Brain in Action*. Oxford: Oxford University Press.

Minshew, N.J. (2001) 'The core deficit in autism and autism spectrum disorders.' *The Journal of Developmental and Learning Disorders 5*, 1, 107–118.

Mitchell, J.P., Brian, J., Zwaigenbaum, L., Szatmari, P., Smith, I. and Bryson, S. (2006) 'Early language and communication development of infants later diagnosed with autism spectrum disorder.' *Journal of Developmental and Behavioral Pediatrics 27*, Suppl. 2, S69–S78.

Mithen, S.J. (1996) *The Prehistory of the Mind: A Search for the Origins of Art, Science and Religion*. London: Thames & Hudson.

Morris, B. (1999) 'New light and insight on an old matter.' *Autism99 Internet Conference Papers*. Available from www.autism99.org, accessed on 12 March 1999.

Mountcastle, V.B. (1997) 'The columnar organization of the neocortex.' *Brain 120*, 701–722.

Mujica-Parodi, L.R., Strey, H.H., Frederick, B., Savoy, R., Cox, D., Botanov, Y., Tolkunov, D., Rubin, D. and Weber, J. (2008) 'Second-hand stress: Neurobiological evidence for a human alarm pheromone.' *Nature Precedings*. Available from http://precedings.nature.com/documents/2561/version/1/files/npre20082561-1.pdf, accessed on 22 March 2010.

Mukhopadhyay, T. (2000) 'My memory.' Accessed at www.cureautismnow.org/tito/memories/my_memory.pdf (site no longer active), on 28 December 2000.

Mukhopadhyay, T. (2008) *How Can I Talk If My Lips Don't Move?: Inside My Autistic Mind.* New York: Arcade Publishing.

Muller, R.A., Behen, M.E., Rothermel, R.D., Chugani, D.C., Muzik, O., Mangner, T.J. and Chugani, H.T. (1999) 'Brain mapping of language and auditory perception in high-functioning autistic adults: A PET study.' *Journal of Autism Developmental Disorders 29*, 19–31.

Neisser, U. and Becklen, R. (1975) 'Selective looking: Attending to visually significant events.' *Cognitive Psychology 7*, 480–494.

Netzer-Pinnick, J. (1998) 'Cover Letter to Sitzman's *The 3rd Approach*.' Available from www.goldenfc.com/articles/sitzman/may25, accessed on 22 March 2010.

Newson, E. (1977) 'Postscript to Lorna Selfe, *Nadia: A Case of Extraordinary Drawing Ability in an Autistic Child.* London: Academic Press.

Noel, D.C. (ed.) (1976) *Reactions to the 'Don Juan' Writings of Carlos Castaneda.* New York: Capricorn Books.

Noll, R. (1983) 'Shamanism and schizophrenia: A state specific approach to the "schizophrenia metaphor" of shamanic states.' *American Ethnologist 10*, 443–459.

Noll, R. (1985) 'Mental imagery cultivation as a cultural phenomenon: The role of visions in shamanism.' *Current Anthropology 26*, 443–461.

O'Connor, N. and Hermelin, B. (1987) 'Visual and graphic abilities of the idiot-savant artist.' *Psychology and Medicine 17*, 1, 79–90.

O'Neill, J. (1999) *Through the Eyes of Aliens: A Book about Autistic People.* London: Jessica Kingsley Publishers.

O'Neill, J. (2003) 'My Experiences Being Autistic.' Available from www.bluepsy.com/jasmine.html, accessed on 5 April 2001.

O'Riordan, M. and Passetti, F. (2006) 'Discrimination in autism within different sensory modalities.' *Journal of Autism and Developmental Disorders 36*, 665–675.

O'Riordan, M.A., Plaisted, K.C., Driver, J. and Baron-Cohen, S. (2001) 'Superior visual search in autism.' *Journal of Experimental Psychology: Human Perception and Performance 27*, 719–730.

Ornitz, E.M. (1969) 'Disorders of perception common to early infantile autism and schizophrenia.' *Comprehensive Psychiatry 10*, 259–274.

Ornitz, E.M. (1974) 'The modulation of sensory input and motor output in autistic children.' *Journal of Autism and Childhood Schizophrenia 4*, 197–215.

Ornitz, E.M. (1983) 'The functional neuroanatomy of infantile autism.' *International Journal of Neuroscience 19*, 85–124.

Ornitz, E.M. (1985) 'Neurophysiology of infantile autism.' *Journal of the American Academy of Child Psychiatry 24*, 251–262.

Ornitz, E.M. (1989) 'Autism at the interface between sensory and information processing.' In G. Dawson (ed.) *Autism: Nature, Diagnosis and Treatment.* New York: Guilford Press.

Ornitz, E.M., Guthrie, D. and Farley, A.J. (1977) 'The early development of autistic children.' *Journal of Autism and Childhood Schizophrenia 7,* 207–229.

Ornitz, E.M., Guthrie, D. and Farley, A.J. (1978) 'The Early Symptoms of Childhood Autism.' In G. Serban (ed.) *Cognitive Deficits in the Development of Mental Illness.* New York: Brunner/Mazel.

Orwell, G. (1949/1987) *Nineteen Eighty-Four.* London: Penguin Books.

Osborn, J. and Derbyshire, S.W.G. (2010) 'Pain sensation evoked by observing injury in others.' *Pain 148,* 2, 268–274.

Pause, B.M., Adolph, D., Prehn-Kristensen, A. and Ferstl, R. (2009) 'Startle response potentiation to chemosensory anxiety signals in socially anxious individuals.' *International Journal of Psychophysiology 74,* 2, 88–92.

Peters, A. and Sethares, C. (1997) 'The organization of double bouquet cells in monkey striate cortex.' *Journal of Neurocytology 26,* 779–797.

Peters, L.G. and Price-Williams, D. (1980) 'Towards an experiential analysis of shamanism.' *American Ethnologist 7,* 398–418.

Pickover, C. (2005) *Sex, Drugs, Einstein, and Elves.* Petaluma, CA: Smart Publications.

Pinker, S. (1994/2000) *The Language Instinct.* New York: Harper Perennial.

Potter, D., Summerfelt, A., Gold, J. and Buchanan, R.W. (2006) 'Review of clinical correlates of P50 sensory gating abnormalities in patients with schizophrenia.' *Schizophrenia Bulletin 32,* 692–700.

Powell, S. (2000) 'Learning about life asocially: The autistic perspective on education.' In S. Powell (ed.) *Helping Children with Autism to Learn.* London: David Fulton Publishers.

Preston, S.D. and de Waal, F.B.M. (2002) 'Empathy: Each is in the right – hopefully, not all in the wrong.' *Behavioral and Brain Science 25,* 1–71.

Pring, L. and Hermelin, B. (2002) 'Numbers and letters: Exploring an autistic savant's unpractised ability.' *Neurocase 8,* 330–370.

Pullum, G.K. (1991) *The Great Eskimo Vocabulary Hoax and Other Irreverent Essays on the Study of Language.* Chicago, IL: University of Chicago Press.

Radin, D. (1998) *The Conscious Universe: The Scientific Truth of Psychic Phenomena.* London: HarperCollins.

Radin, D. (2000) 'Time-reversed human experience: Experimental evidence and implication.' Available from www.emergentmind.org/PDF_files.htm/timereversed. pdf, accessed on 22 March 2010.

Raghanti, M.A., Spocter, M.A., Butti, C., Hof, P.R. and Sherwood, C.C. (2010) 'A comparative perspective on minicolumns and inhibitory GABAergic interneurons in the neocortex.' *Frontiers in Neuroanatomy 4,* 3, 1–10.

Ramachandran, V.S. (2003) *The Emerging Mind: The BBC Reith Lectures.* London: Profile Books.

Rensink, A.R. (1998) 'Mindsight: Visual sensing without seeing.' *Investigative Ophthalmology and Visual Science 39,* 631.

Rensink, R.A. (2000a) 'The dynamic representation of scenes.' *Visual Cognition 7,* 17–42.

Rensink, R.A. (2000b) 'Seeing, sensing, and scrutinizing.' *Vision Research 40*, 1469–1487.

Rensink, R.A. (2004) 'Visual sensing without seeing.' *Psychological Science 15*, 1, 27–32.

Rensink, R.A., O'Regan, J.K. and Clark, J.J. (1997) 'To see or not to see: The need for attention to perceive changes in scenes.' *Psychological Science 8*, 368–373.

Rhine, L.E. (1969) 'Case study review.' *Journal of Parapsychology 33*, 228–266.

Ridington, R. (1979) 'Sequence and hierarchy in cultural experience: Phases and the moment of transformation.' *Anthropology Humanism Quarterly 4*, 4, 2–10.

Ridington, R. (1990) *Little Bit Know Something: Stories in the Language of Anthropology.* Iowa City, IA: University of Iowa Press.

Rimland, B. (1964) *Infantile Autism: The Syndrome and Its Implications for a Neural Therapy of Behavior.* New York: Appleton Century Crofts.

Ritz, B., Ascherio, A., Checkoway, H., Marder, K.S., Nelson, L.M., Rocca, W., Ross, G.W., Strickland, D., Van Den Eeden, S.K. and Gorell, J. (2007) 'Pooled Analysis of Tobacco Use and Risk of Parkinson Disease.' *Archives of Neurology 64*, 7, 990–997.

Robbins, I. (2008) 'Total Isolation.' BBC documentary, 22 January.

Rosen, R. (1985) *Anticipatory Systems.* New York: Pergamon Press.

Rosenblum, L.D., Wuestefeld, A. and Anderson, K. (1996) 'Auditory reachability: An affordance approach to the perception of distance.' *Ecological Psychology 8*, 1–24.

Rosenblum, L.D., Wuestefeld, A. and Saldaña, H. (1993) 'Auditory looming perception: Influences on anticipator judgments.' *Perception 22*, 1467–1482.

Rubenstein, J.L.R. and Merzenich, M.M. (2003) 'Model of autism: Increased ratio of excitation/inhibition in key neural systems.' *Genes, Brain and Behavior 2*, 255–267.

Rutter, M., Andersen-Wood, L., Beckett, C., Bredenkamp, D., Castle, J., Groothues, C., Kreppner, J., Keaveney, L., Lord, C. and O'Connor, T. (1999) 'Quasi-autistic patterns following global privation.' *Journal of Child Psychology and Psychiatry 40*, 537–549.

Ryzl, M. (1966) 'A method of training in ESP.' *International Journal of Parapsychology 8*, p.4.

Sacks, O. (1995) *An Anthropologist on Mars.* London: Picador.

Samuel, G. (2009) 'Autism and meditation: Some reflections.' *Journal of Religion, Disability and Health 13*, 85–93.

Sapir, E. (1929/1949) *Selected Writing in Language, Culture, and Personality* (ed.) D.G. Mandelbaum. Berkeley, CA: University of California Press.

Schacter, D.L. (1987) 'Implicit memory: History and current status.' *Journal of Experimental Psychology: Learning, Memory and Cognition 13*, 501–518.

Schmidt, S., Schneider, R., Utts, J. and Walach, H. (2004) 'Distant intentionality and the feeling of being stared at: Two meta-analyses.' *British Journal of Psychology 95*, 235–247.

Schoonmaker, S. (2008) *Predicting Human Behavior.* Accessed at www.sheilaschoonmaker. com (site no longer active without password), on 4 October 2008.

Selfe, L. (1977) *Nadia: A Case of Extraordinary Drawing Ability in an Autistic Child.* London: Academic Press.

Selfe, L. (1983) *Normal and Anomalous Representational Drawing Ability in Children.* London: Academic Press

Selfe, L. (1985) 'Anomalous Drawing Development: Some Clinical Studies.' In N.H. Freeman and M.V. Cox (eds) *Visual Order: The Nature and Development of Pictorial Representation.* Cambridge: Cambridge University Press.

Shah, A. and Frith, U. (1993) 'Why do autistic individuals show superior performance on the block design task?' *Child Psychology and Psychiatry 34,* 1351–1364.

Sheldrake, R. (1999) *Dogs that Know When Their Owners Are Coming Home.* London: Hutchinson.

Sheldrake, R. (2004) *The Sense of Being Stared At and Other Aspects of the Extended Mind.* London: Arrow Books Ltd.

Sheldrake, R., McKenna, T. and Abraham, R. (2005) *The Evolutionary Mind: Conversations on Science, Imagination and Spirit.* Rhinebeck, NY: Monkfish Book Publishing.

Shermer, M. (2006) In J. Brockman (ed.) *What We Believe But Cannot Prove: Today's Leading Thinkers on Science in the Age of Creativity.* London: Pocket Books.

Shiffrin, R.M. (1988) 'Attention.' In R.C. Atkinson, R.J. Herrnstein, G. Lindzey and R.D. Luce (eds) *Stevens' Handbook of Experimental Psychology: Vol. 2. Learning and Cognition.* New York: Wiley.

Shore, S. (2003) 'Life on and slightly to the right of the Autism Spectrum.' *Exceptional Parent Magazine,* October, 85–90.

Siegel, D.J., Minshew, N.J. and Goldstein, G. (1996) 'Wechsler IQ profiles in diagnosis of high-functioning autism.' *Journal of Autism and Developmental Disorders 26,* 389–406.

Siikala, A. (1978) 'The Rite Technique of the Siberian Shaman.' *(Fellows Folklore Communications 220),* Helsinki: Academia Scientiarium Ethologica.

Silberberg, G., Gupta, A., and Markram, H. (2002) 'Stereotypy in neocortical microcircuits.' *Trends in neurosciences, 25,* 5, 227–230.

Silverman, D. (1975) *Reading Castaneda.* London: Routledge and Kegan Paul.

Silverman, J. (1967) 'Shamanism and acute schizophrenia.' *American Anthropologist 69,* 21–31.

Simons, D. and Chabris, C (1999) 'Gorilla in Our Midst.' *Perception 28,* 1059–1074.

Sinclair, J. (1992) 'Bridging the Gap: An Inside View of Autism.' In E. Schopler and G.B. Mesibov (eds) *High-functioning Individuals with Autism.* New York: Plenum Press.

Sitzman, Y.M. (Undated) *The Religious Ramifications.* Available from www.goldenfc.com/articles/sitzman/rrfc.htm (site no longer active), accessed on 21 October 2007.

Sitzman, Y.M. (1998) *The 3rd Approach.* Available from www.goldenfc.com/articles/sitzman/may25, accessed on 22 March 2010.

Smith, I.M. and Bryson, S.E. (2007) 'Gesture imitation in autism: II. Symbolic gestures and pantomimed object use.' *Cognitive Neuropsychology 24,* 679–700.

Snyder, A.W. (1996) 'Breaking mindset.' *Keynote address 'The Mind's New Science'.* Cognitive Science Miniconference, Macquarie University, 14 November. Available from www.centreforthemind.com/publications/Breaking_Mindset.cfm, accessed on 22 March 2010.

Snyder, A.W. (1997) 'Autistic artists give clues to cognition.' *Perception 26,* 93–6.

Snyder, A.W (2001) 'Paradox of the savant mind.' *Nature 413,* 251–252.

Snyder, A.W. (2004) 'Autistic genius?' *Nature 428,* 470–471.

Snyder, A.W., Bahramali, H., Hawker, T. and Mitchell, D.J. (2006) 'Savant-like numerosity skills revealed in normal people by magnetic pulses.' *Perception 35*, 837–845.

Snyder, A.W., Bossomaier, T. and Mitchell, J.D. (2004) 'Concept formation: "Object" attributes dynamically inhibited from conscious awareness.' *Journal of Integrative Neuroscience 3*, 1, 31–46.

Snyder, A.W. and Mitchell, J.D. (1999) 'Is interger arithmetic fundamental to mental processing?: The mind's secret arithmetic.' *Proceedings of the Royal Society of London 266*, 587–92.

Snyder, A.W., Mulcahy, E., Taylor, J.L., Mitchell, D.J., Sachdev, P. and Gandevia, S.C. (2003) 'Savant-like skills exposed in normal people by suppressing the left front-temporal lobe.' *Journal of Integrative Neuroscience 2*, 149–158.

Snyder, A.W. and Thomas, M. (1997) 'Autistic artists give clues to cognition.' *Perception 26*, 93–96.

Sonnby-Borgström, M. (2002) 'The facial expression says more than words. Is emotional "contagion" via facial expression the first step toward empathy?' *Lakartidningen 99*, 1438–1442.

Spicer, D. (1998) 'Self-awareness in living with Asperger syndrome.' *Asperger Syndrome Conference Papers*, Vasteras, Sweden, 12–13 March.

Steklis, H.D. and Harnad, S. (1976) 'From Hand to Mouth: Some Critical Stages in the Evolution of Language.' In S. Harnad, H.D. Steklis and J. Lancaster (eds) *Origin and Evolution of Language and Speech. Annals of the New York Academy of Sciences 280*, 445–455.

Stern, D.N. (1985) *The Interpersonal World of the Infant: A View from Psychoanalysis and Developmental Psychology.* New York: Basic Books.

Stern, D.N. (1994) 'One way to build a clinically relevant baby.' *Infant Mental Health Journal 15*, 9–25.

Stillman, W. (2006) *Autism and the God Connection: Redefining the Autistic Experience through Extraordinary Accounts of Spiritual Giftedness.* Naperville, IL: Sourcebooks.

Surakka, V. and Hietanen, J.K. (1998) 'Facial and emotional reactions to Duchenne and non-Duchenne smiles.' *International Journal of Psychophysiology 29*, 23–33.

Szalavitz, M. (2009) 'Asperger's theory does about-face.' *Healthzone.ca.* Available from www.healthzone.ca/health/articlePrint/633688, accessed on 22 March 2010.

Tammet, D. (2006) *Born on a Blue Day: A Memoir of Asperger's and an Extraordinary Mind.* London: Hodder and Stoughton.

Tammet, D. (2009) *Embracing the Wide Sky: A Tour across the Horizons of the Mind.* London: Hodder and Stoughton.

Tanguay, P.E. and Edwards, R. (1982) 'Electrophysiological studies of autism: The whisper of the bang.' *Journal of Autism and Developmental Disorders 12*, 2, 177–184.

Tantam, D. (1988) 'Lifelong eccentricity and social isolation. Psychiatric, social, and forensic aspects.' *British Journal of Psychiatry 153*, 777–782.

Tantam, D. (2009) *Can the World Afford Autistic Spectrum Disorders?: Nonverbal Communication, Asperger Syndrome and the Interbrain.* London: Jessica Kingsley Publishers.

Taylor, D. (2004) *Think Cat: An Owner's Guide to Feline Psychology.* London: Cassell Illustrated.

Thompson, L.M. (1950) *Culture in Crisis*. New York: Harper.

Trevarthen, C. and Aitken, K.J. (2001) 'Infant intersubjectivity: Research, theory, and clinical applications.' *Journal of Child Psychology and Psychiatry and Allied Disciplines 42*, 3–48.

Tustin, F. (1974) *Autism and Childhood Psychosis*. London: Hogarth Press.

VanDalen, J.D.T. (1995) 'Autism from within: Looking through the eyes of a mildly afflicted autistic person.' *Link 17*, 11–16.

Velmans, M. (1991) 'Is human information processing conscious?' *Behavioral and Brain Sciences 14*, 651–726.

Volkmar, F.R., Cohen, D.J. and Paul, R. (1986) 'An evaluation of DSM-III criteria for infantile autism.' *Journal of American Academy of Child Psychiatry 25*, 190–197.

Walker, N. and Cantello, J. (eds) (1994) 'You don't have words to describe what I experience.' Available from www.autism.net/infoparent.html, accessed on 24 November 1999.

Warrington, E.K. and Shallice, T. (1984) 'Category-specific semantic impairments.' *Brain 107*, 829–854.

Weiskrantz, L. (1986) *Blindsight: A Case Study and Implications*. Oxford: Oxford University Press.

Weiskrantz, L. (1996) 'Blindsight revisited.' *Current Opinion in Experimental Psychology, 6*, 215–220.

Weiskrantz, L., Warrington, E.K., Sanders, M.D. and Marshall, J. (1974) 'Visual capacity in the hemianopic field following a restricted occipital ablation.' *Brain 97*, 709–728.

White, P.T. (1955) 'The Interpreter: Linguist Plus Diplomat.' *New York Times Magazine, 6* November.

Whorf, B.L. (1940) 'Science and linguistics.' *Technological Review 42*, 229–231, 247–248.

Whorf, B.L. (1941) 'The Relation of Habitual Thought and Behavior to Language.' In L. Spier (ed.) *Language, Culture, and Personality: Essay in Memory of Edward Sapir*. Menasha, WI: Sapir Memorial Publication Fund.

Whorf, B.L. (1950) 'An American Indian model of the universe.' *International Journal of American Linguistics 16*, 67–72.

Whorf, B.L. (1956) *Language, Thought and Reality: Selected Writings*. Cambridge, MA: MIT Press.

Wilbert, J. (1987) *Tobacco and Shamanism in South America*. New Haven, CT: Yale University Press.

Willey, L.H. (1999) *Pretending to Be Normal*. London: Jessica Kingsley Publishers.

Williams, D. (1996) *Autism: An Inside-Out Approach: An Innovative Look at the 'Mechanics' of 'Autism' and Its Developmental 'Cousins'*. London: Jessica Kingsley Publishers.

Williams, D. (1998) *Autism and Sensing: The Unlost Instinct*. London: Jessica Kingsley Publishers.

Williams, D. (1999a) *Like Colour to the Blind: Soul Searching and Soul Finding*. London: Jessica Kingsley Publishers.

Williams, D. (1999b) *Nobody Nowhere: The Remarkable Autobiography of an Autistic Girl*. London: Jessica Kingsley Publishers.

Williams, D. (1999c) *Somebody Somewhere: Breaking Free from the World of Autism.* London: Jessica Kingsley Publishers.

Williams, D. (2003a) *Exposure Anxiety – The Invisible Cage: An Exploration of Self-Protection Responses in the Autism Spectrum and Beyond.* London: Jessica Kingsley Publishers.

Williams, D. (2003b) 'Tinted lenses.' *Autism Today Online Magazine.* Available at www.autismtoday.com/articles/tinted_lenses.htm, accessed on 15 April 2010.

Williams, D. (2005) 'From feral, to author to screenwriter.' Available from www.autismtoday.com/articles/From-Feral.asp?name=DonnaWilliams, accessed on 22 March 2010.

Williams, D. (2007) 'Peripheral vision in some people on the autism spectrum.' Available from http://blog.donnawilliams.net/2007/03/05, accessed on 22 March 2010.

Williams, E.I.F. (1970) *Editorial Introduction* to A.H. Maslow *Religions, Values, and Peak-Experiences.* New York: Penguin.

Wing, L. (1972) 'The handicaps of autistic children.' *Communication,* June, 6–8.

Winkelman, M. (1986) 'Trance states: A theoretical model and cross-cultural analysis.' *Ethos 14,* 174–204.

Winnicott, D.W. (1960) 'Ego Distortion in Terms of True and False Self.' In M.R. Khan (ed.) *The Maturational Processes and the Facilitating Environment: Studies in the Theory of Emotional Development.* New York: International Universities Press.

Winnicott, D.W. (1963) 'Communicating and Not Communicating Leading to a Study of Certain Opposites.' In M.R. Khan (ed.) *The Maturational Processes and the Fascilitating Environment: Studies in the Theory of Emotional Development.* New York: International Universities Press.

Witchel, A. (1997) 'Interview: "At Lunch with Marc Salem"', *New York Times,* 11 December 1997.

Wolf, F.A. (1998) 'The timing of conscious experience: A causality-violating, two-valued, transactional interpretation of subjective antedating and spatial-temporal projection.' *Journal of Scientific Exploration 12,* 4, 511–542.

Wolfe, J.M. (1999) 'Inattentional amnesia.' In V. Coltheart (ed.) *Fleeting Memories.* 71–94. Cambridge, MA: MIT Press.

Zeki, S. (1992) 'The visual image in the mind and brain.' *Scientific American 267,* 3, 69–76.

SUBJECT INDEX

AUTHOR INDEX

38833361R00125

Printed in Great Britain
by Amazon